Callanetics

for Your Back

Other Avon Books by
Callan Pinckney

CALLANETICS

CALLANETICS COUNTDOWN:
30 DAYS TO A BEAUTIFUL BODY

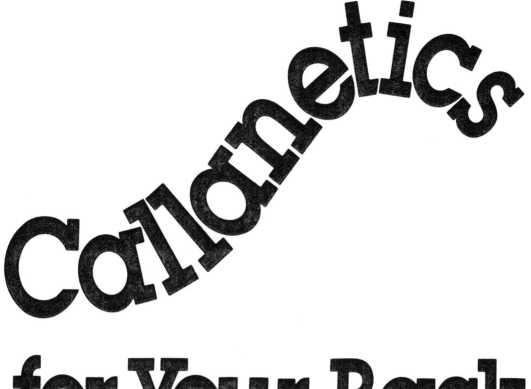

Callanetics
for Your Back

CALLAN PINCKNEY

with

BARBARA FRIEDLANDER MEYER

Research and technical assistance
by Nancy Keith Gerard, OTR

Photographs by Stuart M. Gross

Illustrations by Nazan Akyavas

AVON BOOKS ◢◣ NEW YORK

AVON BOOKS
A division of
The Hearst Corporation
1350 Avenue of the Americas
New York, New York 10019

First Avon Trade Books Printing: June 1990

AVON TRADEMARK REG. U.S. PAT. OFF. AND IN OTHER COUNTRIES, MARCA REGISTRADA, HECHO EN U.S.A.

Printed in the U.S.A.

CW 10 9 8 7 6 5 4 3

To my sister Jane

When life deals you incredible hardships, you are always able to smile like the radiant morning sun and still have the inner strength to put on lipstick.

Thank you for teaching me the gentle, giving power of a smile.

A Note of Caution

The exercises, instructions, and advice presented in this book are in no way intended as a substitute for medical counseling. Consult your doctor before beginning this or any other regimen of exercise. The author and publisher of this book disclaim any liability or loss in connection with the exercises and advice herein.

Pregnant women in the first trimester should not do the abdominal exercises on pages 112 to 120. These exercises are much too powerful to be performed during pregnancy.

Acknowledgments

To Dr. Patrick Luongo and Dr. Ron Schmeltzer

Thanks for being on call twenty-four hours a day for advice and demonstrations. But most of all, thank you for your concern for the continuing good health of the readers of this book.

My deepest appreciation to the following people who served as models for the photographs:

Cynthia Birdwell
Lillian Gerard
Nancy Gerard
Arnold Meyer
Lori Shild
Randy Smith
Irwin Trzciak

Endorsements

In keeping with Callan's intention of providing information on the variety of disciplines involved in back care, the following are remarks from some representative practioners:

Reuben S. Ingber, M.D., Physiatrist, New York City: "What distinguishes Callan's method is her balanced approach, emphasizing stretching and neuromuscular coordination while also strengthening the deep, posture muscles. This will develop a more balanced tone throughout the musculoskeletal system, while avoiding possible injury, so frequently encountered when undertaking an exercise program. The posture muscles, the deepest layer of muscles, are important in joint stabilization. Maintaining them in their most relaxed state (stretching), then strengthening them by slow controlled movements, will help avoid the stress syndromes and excess joint compression problems. Further, this can be used as a springboard for safe participation in sports and recreational activities. I endorse this method from a medical vantage point.

"One word of caution, for those in acute pain. I would suggest a medical evaluation prior to undertaking any exercise program."

Dr. Pasquale Luongo, Chiropractor, New York City: What a relief to read a book about the back which is comprehensible to the layman. I found it adventurous, entertaining, funny, and—best of all—accurate. This book is a must for people with back problems. It is filled with practical information, encouragements, and a deep empathy for the difficulties others may have. It also provides excellent suggestions for approaches people can take to help themselves. I can recommend this book enthusiastically to all my patients.

Liz Henry, Registered Physical Therapist, Dance medicine specialist working with the New York City Ballet, and also in private prac-

tice: I feel Callan's regimen can be very helpful in most cases of back pain due to postural dysfunction. Her suggestions and advice are very sound. Particularly useful is the information in the Everyday Exercises chapter, and the truth about harmful exercises in [the chapter] Stay Away from These.

Dr. Harold Stephen Solomon, Hypertension Specialist; author, Beat The Odds, *Boston, Mass.:* Callan Pinckney seems to have written a back book that makes a great deal of sense to me. I was particularly attracted to her ideas about stretching. In my experience, most personal exercise injuries are a result of failure to adequately prepare muscles by stretch and warm-up. I wonder if her penchant for slow, small movements comes from being from the South, where we all moved slowly.

Alexis Phillips, Instructor of Massage and Clinic Supervisor, Swedish Institute, New York City, and Co-Director, Soma seminars and workshops in massage: "Callan is allowing people who are suffering from back problems alternative modalities. She is not taking a strict position and saying there is only one way. This is very helpful, particularly because it makes the person rightly question before pursuing a course."

Foreword

Callan and I have been friends for many years, since she returned to the United States after her eleven-year sojourn around the world.

She often tells me that I was the first American who could understand her and with whom she could communicate. Because she had missed the sixties in America, she felt she was in a sort of time warp. She spoke with an English accent, which was not an affectation but which people thought might be, given the fact that she was American. The United States seemed like a strange country and she was awed by everyone and everything she saw, like a child lost in a toy store. I thought she was delightful and I would marvel at all her colorful stories about her adventures.

One of the first things that impressed me about Callan was her exceptional body and her fantastic legs. So I became one of her early students, even though I hated any kind of exercise. She used to come to my house, where we exercised on the portable barre she'd bring with her and set up in the only available place—my closet. It was all very makeshift but it worked. My body shaped up faster and better than ever before in my life; and my chronic neck and back problems improved greatly. When she moved up in the world (literally) to her high-rise studio, I naturally followed.

Much of Callan's success as a teacher can be credited to her remarkable intuition. I saw it at work many times in classes where she would provide a particular motion or encouraging phrase that a person needed, or hit upon the cause of a particular problem just by observing the way someone held himself. Yet I had no idea of the extent of this gift until we worked on this book. She constantly expounded theories and ideas, which would later be corroborated by hard facts. One example of this was her story about Indian women massaging their babies (see page 154). To me, it was a touching anecdote, but no more than that. Then, months later, I came across an article in a professional journal that went into great length about the scientifically proved therapeutic benefits of massage for babies. Her intuition is just one aspect of Callan that makes her *sui generis*. She is in a class by herself, and so it should come as no surprise that this book is unlike any other book on the back. I knew it would be, which was one of many reasons I was so excited about working on it.

One of my research tasks was to accompany her to all sorts of exercise and body movement classes. I would *walk* through the exercises as she had trained me to do, rather than actually attempting them right away. She, on the other hand, wanting to personally experience anything she wrote about, deliberately did not follow her own advice. Consequently, she suffered problems with her neck or back, whereas I remained injury-free.

In the end, however, I was not spared. While I sat for long hours in front of the word processor, Callan made me try out a variety of positions and experimental chairs. The result? One evening, I got up from my chair and went into my first back spasm. It was so excruciating that I was left speechless. Before this happened, in the course of working on this book, I would often think that some of Callan's statements about spasm were too exaggerated to be real. I was concerned that readers might feel the same way and even suggested tempering some of her remarks. But when I had this attack, I turned to my husband in the middle of a sleepness night and told him I was afraid to even move my fingers. All of a sudden, I could hear myself echoing Callan's words, and realized that they were not hyperbole. It was all true. Perhaps I had to go through that pain to become a true believer. Like Callan, I can now speak from first-hand experience, and nothing equals that. I did do the emergency spasm-relief exercise (page 19), and followed Callan's other advice on exercises and helpers. It worked.

There's something for everyone here. Whether you're a chronic back sufferer or someone who wants to prevent ever being one, this book will provide you with what you need to know—and entertain you while doing it.

—*Barbara Friedlander Meyer*

Contents

Foreword 11

Introduction 15

1. Emergency Relief for Spasm 19

2. Choose Your Stretches 23

3. Minnie Mouse's Shoes and Other Foot
   Travesties 47

4. Stretches for a Bad Back 51

5. Everyday Activities 59

6. Everyday Exercises 73

7. Three Stages of Callanetics 83
   Pelvic Wave 88

8. Stay Away from These 139

9. People Helpers 149

10. Power of the Mind 159

11. You're Never Too Young or Too Old 164

12. A Brief Anatomy Lesson 169

13. Some Common Causes of Back Pain 175

14. Other Ways and Means to Relieve Back
    Symptoms 185

Index 191

Introduction

How in the world did I end up writing this book? I presume if I had to choose the primary motives, they would be anger and frustration. I had been teaching body movement since 1972, and up until 1981 maybe one out of twenty students had a history of back problems. Suddenly, starting in 1981, it became fourteen out of twenty new students who were back sufferers. To me, this was a staggering percentage, and one didn't have to be a genius to figure out why. These people were victims of America's radical "injury movement" (supposedly, the fitness movement), and many had been referred to me because my program had produced excellent results for other back sufferers.

All at once, every conversation seemed to include the subject of bad backs. I remember going to a business dinner with ten people, five of whom spent the entire time comparing back problems (and two had a field day competing with each other over whose neck was worse). This was even less than the national average; next to colds, backache is the most common "ailment" in America. Estimates are that 80 percent of the population has back problems, and ninety million dollars are lost each year from absences due to back problems. One insurance company pays out more than a million dollars each day in back-related claims.

After my first book, *Callanetics*, was published, I continued to view television programs, magazines, and books pertinent to my profession. I was very upset to see that many of the popular exercises being demonstrated could still be injurious to even a healthy back. (In 1988 it's still the same story, unfortunately.)

From these experiences, I began to feel the need to make the public aware of the many resources available specifically for protecting and treating the back.

But what really clinched my decision to write a book about the back was the voluminous amount of phone calls and letters I received from people telling me how much *Callanetics* had helped their backs. Many also begged for answers to questions like: What kind of doctor should I go to? What's the difference between this and that technique, and are any of them good for my back? What can I do if one leg is shorter than the other? The questions were practically without end.

Naturally, I did not have all the answers—and I didn't mind admitting that. But it seemed that many back "experts" or self-ordained gurus were saying, "My way is the *only* way." And what we were left with was confusion. All of this verified what I had known instinctively for so many years: People were not getting the kind of information they needed.

In *Callanetics*, I wrote about my physical problems in detail. I have had back trouble all my life, only during my early years I never spoke about it because it wasn't considered in good taste to discuss your ailments with other people. As I had been born with club feet, I had to wear steel braces up to my waist for seven years. When I was twenty-one, I left the United States for a three-month tour of Europe. I returned home eleven years later, after walking around most of the world with a sixty-five-pound rucksack resting on my lower back.

By the time I arrived home, my knees, neck, shoulders, and feet had joined with my back to complete the picture: a perfect wreck! (I did get a lovely reward, though: I knew the location of almost every country in the world, could draw its shape and spell its name correctly; big deal—most have changed their names since!)

I feel the main thrust of a comprehensive back book must be to make you aware of your body by increasing your knowledge. Then you can be in control of protecting and healing it. Awareness of one's body is the master key. Most people carry their bodies from point *A* to point *B*, basically unconscious of the fact that their bodies are their home. You live in your body twenty-four hours a day for all of your life. Yet how often do you think about it that way?

Treating your back entails:

• Investigating different techniques and experimenting so that you can make informed choices.
• Being willing to discipline yourself until something becomes a habit.
• Developing a positive attitude to motivate you and encourage you to succeed.

My own experience with investigation and experimentation involved an enormous amount of research—at least twenty-four books, most by medical doctors; dozen of articles; and many videotapes. The experimentation was particularly grueling because, since I began doing Callanetics years ago, I had been virtually free of back pain (except when I did something dumb). Now, if I followed all the advice found in my research, I would have to regress to certain habits that I was reasonably sure might start the whole cycle of back pain again, or worse, a recurrence of spasms.

But I wanted to experiment to make it possible for you to avoid any kind of injurious experimentation. Naturally, few back problems are identical, but there are certain principles that apply to all.

You certainly should not feel obligated to experiment. If you choose to, you should be extremely careful about what you do, in order to avoid possible injury. After all, there were certain things I felt I *had* to do; you do not. On the other hand, don't take my word or anyone else's when it comes to your body—that's part of taking responsibility. It is my wish that you make informed choices. If I had to single out the major aim of this book, it would be to provide you with enough alternatives and information to make safe choices that work for *you*.

I'm fanatic about my readers being able to understand the subject. The best information in the world is useless if you can't understand it. Many books on the back are incomprehensible to the lay person. They are written by people who sincerely want to convey information but, in a sense, speak another language. Their technical vocabulary is not ours. It took me eight hours to read twenty-six pages of a book written by a doctor for general publication—and I knew what he was talking about! I think readers don't really care what the name of a particular bone is, such as *ischial tuberosities*; you only need to know that it's one of the sit bones. For this reason, I took particular care to ensure that the vocabulary in this book is as clear as possible.

Let's start with the subject of pain. It seems logical to associate back problems with pain. Although it is not always true, back pain usually signals back trouble, and it is important for you to get a correct diagnosis. On the other hand, trouble with the back or neck may manifest itself as pain in other areas such as knees, ankles, calves; or as headaches, indigestion, numbness in fingers and toes. So how can we evaluate a condition on the basis of pain? Pain affects the way you function, the way you look, and your whole attitude about your life and the world. Yet for many people pain is a fact of life that they take for granted and feel they can do nothing about. Nonsense!

Sometimes pain can be a wonderful opportunity to understand your body and your psyche. I had students who were not even aware of the extent of their chronic pain until they learned through the exercises in class how they could eliminate it. It was only then that they realized that they did not have to suffer any longer. After this experience, they were willing to make very simple changes in their life-styles in order to protect their backs (such as being conscious of not slumping over while sitting). In this way, pain can be used a preventive measure.

And prevention is essential to back care. Even if you are one of those rare people who has never had a backache, you should still protect that area, which is—in every way—the spine of your body. Sometimes, back problems can be present without your knowing. For instance, I was told by a back specialist that it takes 80 percent of a nerve to be pinched before you feel it. Because the spine has so much cushioning to protect it from shocks and jolts, you may have serious problems before you begin to experience any pain or even discomfort.

Why wait to have back problems before doing the best things you can to prevent them? You can develop awareness of how to move your body and learn the right kind of exercise *for you*. This book gives you many opportunities to choose a body motion program. Whatever you do, you must do it regularly: *Inactivity is the curse of the back sufferer*. Like brushing your teeth, a back care regimen must become second nature. This is not meant to imply that you have to resign yourself to boredom and drudgery. It may, however, require some new self-discipline—such as giving up the most entertaining and "fun" exercises if they do not serve you. But the exercises that do serve you can also be fun, because they are helping you to feel better, get stronger, and learn to alleviate your back pain.

The kind of physical discipline I advocate builds inner strength, self-respect, and a wonderful sense of accomplishment. In my fifteen years of teaching, none of my students has even sustained an injury. The main reason is my technique which, stated simply, is *no impact*; with it, people can obtain extremely fast results in tightening their body while learning to protect their back at the same time.

Another reason is that my students learn the art of discipline, from the first class. I insist that when they begin, they work in *triple slow motion*—imagine slowing down a slow-motion movie—which enables them to become aware of everything that's happening with their body. The combination of my specific motions done in triple slow motion is a commonsense approach to preventing injuries. With these techniques, students can immediately learn to work at their own pace, not that of the student next to them, or mine.

You must develop a positive attitude. This idea is discussed at greater length in the chapter called Power of the Mind (see page 159). Your well-being depends as much on your willingness to succeed as the method you use to get there. Let's face it—all of us feel negative about our body some of the time (and some of us all of the time!). We also usually loathe doing anything about it. It's a real struggle to combat this force, yet we *can* get past it—even if we have to make it a game, even if we have to fantasize about being our favorite actor or dancer in order to get through the exercise routine. I know that regardless of how much I resist, I will have to do my exercises consistently for my back for the rest of my life. So whenever I need a boost to continue, I can always call up my favorite vision: I am the captain of a pirate ship, draped in clinging ivory satin, swinging across on a rope, with a Turkish knife between my teeth, to rescue Erroll Flynn. I will sweep him off the enemy deck with one arm as we swing back to safety—all of which I accomplish because my back is now so strong.

1.

Emergency Relief for Spasm

T his chapter is specifically designed to assist in quickly relieving a spasm. Although there is controversy among practitioners on this issue, it has been my firsthand experience that muscle spasms respond positively to immediate attention. So don't be afraid to try it; I feel the longer your muscle remains in spasm, the longer it may take to heal.

The following stretches work like traction by using the weight and strength of your body, instead of that dreadful hospital pulley system that can keep you immobile for weeks.

Even if you have access to a barre for hanging, I recommend that you don't use it at first if you have any lower back problems. Instead, begin by using a sink, countertop, table, sofa, or other stable surface (one that won't fall if you pull too hard). Doing the exercises this way will provide a substitute for hanging from a barre, allowing you to use the stretch to its fullest potential at a beginner's level.

NOTE: Many exercises in this book involve doing what I call the pelvic wave. Although this is discussed in detail on pages 88 to 94, a brief explanation is appropriate here.

The pelvic wave can be done either lying down or standing. Very gently and slowly, tighten your buttocks and, in triple slow motion, curl your pelvis up, aiming it into the navel. Be conscious of the beautiful stretch in your spine. The pelvic wave causes you to automatically tighten your abdominal muscles, inner and front thighs, and buttocks muscles. It will make you aware of how a delicate, small motion can do such important work in protecting the back.

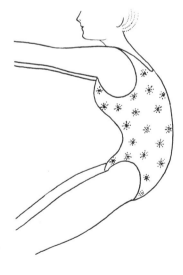

> The exercises in this chapter must be done
> in triple slow motion. Please see page 87.

EMERGENCY SPASM RELIEF #1

1. Stand in front of a chair, counter, table, or other piece of stable furniture that is a comfortable height for your arms to reach. Stand an arm's length away, feet a hip-width apart. Stretch arms out, hold on to edge with both hands, and bend knees. Keep head centered between arms.

2. Holding on to edge, pull torso away from counter, aiming buttocks down. Keep spine straight; do not let buttocks go lower than knees. Do pelvic wave. Hold for a count of 5 to 10. Breathe naturally and feel the stretch all along your spine, shoulders, and lower back.

3. To come out of position, still holding on, maintain pelvic wave; then, trying to keep shoulders rounded, gently stand up, curling up pelvis even more.

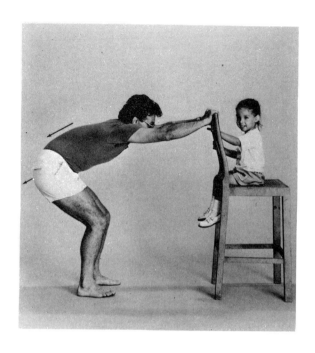

EMERGENCY SPASM RELIEF #2

1. Stand in front of chair, counter, table, or other stable piece of furniture that is at a comfortable height for your arms to reach. Stand an arm's length away, feet a hip-width apart. Stretch arms out, hold on to edge with both hands and bend knees. Keep head centered between arms.

2. Holding on to edge, pull torso away from counter, aiming buttocks away from counter (don't let buttocks go lower than knees). Stretch spine. Hold for a count of 5 to 10. Breathe naturally and feel the stretch all along your spine, shoulders, and lower back.

3. Gently bring right hip forward and then up toward ceiling, trying to get it as high as possible. You can let your heel come up off the floor if necessary. Hold for a count of 5 to 10.

4. Gently release right hip. Repeat with left hip. Return to center.

5. Still holding on, do pelvic wave; then gently stand up, trying to round shoulders and curl up pelvis even more.

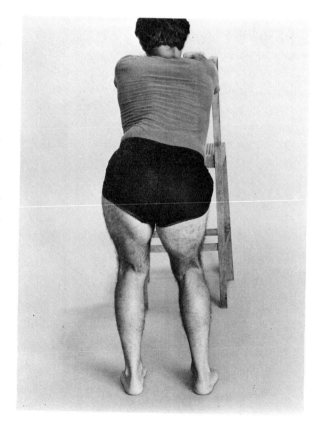

NOTE: If it is too difficult to bring hip forward and up, you can move it directly to the side.

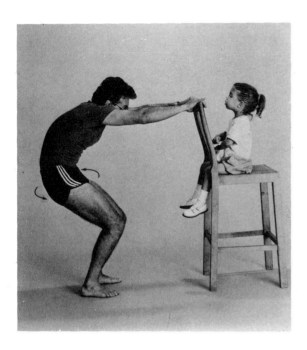

EMERGENCY SPASM RELIEF #3

1. Stand in front of a counter at arm's length, feet a hip-width apart. Hold on to edge with both hands and bend knees. Stretch entire torso away from counter, making back as straight as possible. Keep head level with arms and relaxed. Hold for a count of 10. (**Caution:** If you cannot keep your back straight, return to Exercises 1 and 2. Under no circumstances should the back be arched in this exercise.)

2. With knees still bent, aim buttocks away from counter (as in #1). Very gently, in slow motion practice pelvic wave (curling pelvis up and releasing it). (Do not stick buttocks out when releasing it.) You will not have the range of movement possible with the standard pelvic wave because of the torso's position, but it will still contribute to loosening your lower back.

3. Rotate pelvis in a circle 3 times in each direction, using triple slow motion. Do not stick out buttocks. Still holding on to counter, tighten buttocks, curl up pelvis, and release hands as you slowly come to a standing position, one vertebra at a time.

2.

Choose Your Stretches

Stretching is not a luxury—it is absolutely essential that you do some form of it every day. Muscles shrink back and tighten up if they are not stretched regularly. A high percentage of all sports injuries could be averted by properly stretching muscles, to keep them flexible. That goes for *all* types of exercise; you just won't be able to handle the strains and stress of exercising if your muscles are too tight. Throughout the day, you create physical stress from performing activities in awkward postural positions (for instance, certain jobs or sports use one side of the body predominantly), as well as mental and emotional stress. Stretching leads to relaxation, increased flexibility, better circulation and balance. It helps counteract the effects of tension; it keeps joints lubricated, which helps prevent stiffness of joints by increasing your range of movement in all muscles and tendons. In my opinion, it even helps to slow down the aging process. Possibly most important is that it makes you feel more alive, and for this reason you'll want to continue it. Measure your stretch by how it feels, not by how far you can go. Because it's so individual, stretching ability can vary from day to day. Some days you will be more limber than others. Never try to push yourself on a stiff day to reach the level you were on the day before. A good way to test whether you're overdoing a stretch is how you feel coming out of it: It shouldn't be difficult to return to your original position. Remember, never stretch to the point of being uncomfortable.

There's no limit to the opportunities you have to stretch. You can stretch in small, inconspicuous ways while waiting for a bus, or during a coffee break instead of drinking the coffee; or you can do a whole program when you have the time. I was amazed, while on my book and video tours, when so many people told me they were starting to use their time in the evening to exercise; it was an activity they could do for themselves and, at the same time, be with their children. Use stretching techniques in a tense situation, such as when you're stuck in traffic; instead of having a severe anxiety attack, sitting on the horn, cursing everyone in sight, wanting to rip apart the poor person in front of you and feeling totally helpless, turn this impossible situation into a blessed time for you to do the neck stretches. During my long walk around the world, on the rare occasions when I was freed of my ''house'' (backpack), I would grab the nearest tree limb, give a big yell, pretend I was Tarzan (not Jane!), and stretch to my pathetic limit.

Although there are differences of opinion on the prime time to stretch, I concur with stretching both at night to prevent stiffness the next morning; and in the morning to undo the stiffness that may set in while sleeping. Choose whichever time suits you; any time of the day is wonderful as long as you do it. Regardless of how active you are, or how much you use your body, stretching is a necessity.

Stretching is an individual activity. You should not compete, either with yourself or others, or allow another person, who may not know the limit of your flexibility at the time, to help you. I don't like using muscles against another force or prop. This could result in injury. Use only the strength of your own muscles; only they know what they are or are not capable of doing. Everyone is naturally limited by factors of heredity, age, and physical condition. For example, if you were born with tight or loose ligaments, you can't change the structure; but you can adapt it to your activities. Also, there are no shortcuts to reaching *your* maximum stretchability; it happens in its own time, and you can't force it without danger of injury. Being in control of your body means knowing that your muscles are telling you what they can do; you don't tell them. Just as in contracting, when you can do only a certain amount of repetitions before the muscle fatigues, you can only stretch so far before there is pain and the muscle could tear. Some of my pet peeves are programs which outline your stretching goals and have you score yourself. Supposedly, you are to progress at the rate determined by the scorecard makers. I have known people who, because they weren't able to stretch for a few days, tried to make it up all at one time. You don't win at this game—it's better to fail the test and stay out of the doctor's office. It's really all right to take a day off and rest—more will be lost than gained if you push yourself too hard.

The stretch reflex is a mechanism which is an intrinsic part of the body designed to protect the muscles. When the fibers are being overstretched, an automatic signal is sent to tell the muscles to contract before injury occurs. If you stretch too far, or do vigorous bouncing movements, you activate the stretch reflex, thereby tightening the very muscles you are trying to stretch.

There are three main stretching techniques: ballistic (bouncing), static, and contract-relax. Ballistic movements are no longer recommended because they activate the stretch reflex. Static stretching involves stretching to the point where you feel a pull in the muscle and then holding it at that point for a specified time (until you feel the tension release). Contract-relax involves stretching a muscle to its point of stretch, applying resistance in the opposite direction, holding for about three seconds, and then resting for one second. Then you stretch the muscle even farther to a new point.

My stretches are mostly static rather than contract-relax. I dislike using any force other than your own strength. However, if you prefer to move a bit, you will notice that I give you the option of moving very, very slightly (no more than $\frac{1}{16}$ inch). You may hold a stretch for 60 seconds, which is about how long it takes for a muscle to adjust and then relax. Or, if you wish, you may hold the stretch for a count of 10 to 30 (depending on your ability) and move $\frac{1}{16}$ inch for as many times as I stipulate.

Most of the following stretches call for you to stretch one side of the body at a time. This is particularly advantageous because the two sides of the body are not the same; one side is usually more limber than the other. For this reason, you should do more stretching on the less flexible side, especially if you've been in spasm on that side. People usually work the more stretched side first and harder, rushing through and giving less time to the weaker side, which really needs more attention.

Before you begin the following stretches, here are some very important points to remember:

1. Warm up in order to raise the body's temperature and make the muscles more pliable; warm muscles make stretching easier and safer. You may run or walk fast in place for about five minutes or take a warm shower, or whatever else fits into your life-style. Realistically, many people do not have time to warm up. If this is the case, you must be *extra* careful not to overstretch or strain.
2. Warm up before stretching and after any vigorous activity.
3. Move very slowly through the entire stretch, including coming out of it. Think of moving in triple slow motion: Whether lying down or standing up, pretend your body is melting into the floor. Every stretch should feel comfortable; never do it to the point of pain.
4. Breathing technique is not so important as long as you remember to do it! You may breathe naturally, or deeply and slowly, exhaling completely before inhaling again.
5. Feel the stretch in the muscles themselves, not in joints, tendons, or ligaments.
6. Keep your state of mind relaxed and positive. Be patient. Think beautiful thoughts; visualize your dreams coming true.
7. If you're new to stretching or you haven't stretched in a while, allow yourself an extra dose of patience.

In addition to the following stretches, see Stretches for Bad Backs and Three Stages of Callanetics for other stretching exercises.

Be careful! This is a powerful stretch. If you are not ready for it, you cause strain or discomfort. Do not do this and the following exercise (Towel #II) if you have shoulder problems.

SHOULDERS/CHEST

NOTE: The following two exercises can also be done seated.

Towel I

1. Stand with legs a hip-width apart; back straight; head, neck, and shoulders relaxed. Bend knees, tighten buttocks, curl up pelvis (pelvic wave).

2. Hold a towel, rope, or other flexible material (not a broom or pole) with both hands in front of you. In triple slow motion, to a count of 10 to 15, bring over head and behind back as low as possible. Keep elbows bent in the beginning; after a period of time you may straighten them for a greater stretch, but do not force.

3. Return to original position to a count of 15 to 30.

NOTE: When you are comfortable with maximum stretching point, you can hold it for a count of 60; if you wish, after a count of 15 to 30, move arms up and down no more than ¹⁄₁₆ inch, 5 to 10 times.

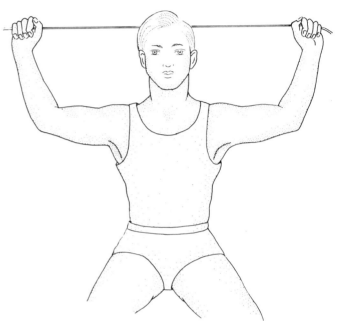

> *Stretches chest, shoulders, upper arms*
>
> Do not *thrust head out; arch lower back; stick out buttocks, tense neck and shoulders; force motion*

Towel II

1. Stand with legs a hip-width apart; back straight; head, neck, and shoulders relaxed. Bend knees, tighten buttocks, curl up pelvis (pelvic wave).

2. With right hand, drop towel behind back, lifting right elbow as high above shoulder as possible. Bring left hand to reach behind you, and move it up as high as possible (without forcing) to grab towel. Gently pull and hold for a count of 15 to 30.

3. Release slowly and repeat on other side.

> *Stretches upper arms, shoulders, chest*
> Do not *force motion; arch lower back; stick out buttocks*

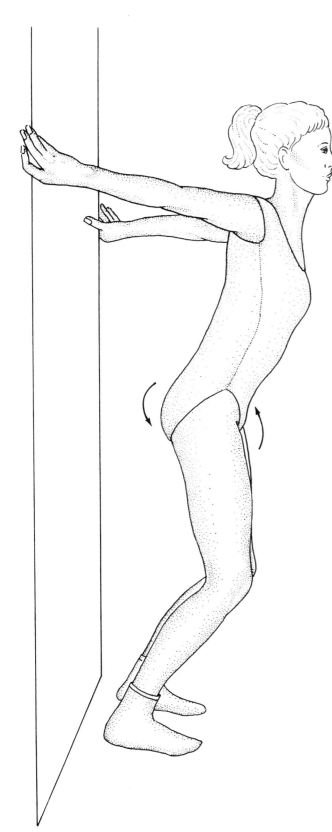

Door

1. Stand in front of doorway, with your back to it. Bring arms behind you at about shoulder height and hold on to door frame. Move body forward until arms are straight (about 1 to 1½ feet). Bend knees and keep feet facing forward.

2. Lean torso forward as much as possible (making sure chin is pulled in); tighten buttocks and curl up pelvis (pelvic wave). Hold for a count of 60. Or, if you wish, after a count of 15 to 30, move torso forward and back no more than ¹⁄₁₆ inch, 5 to 10 times. When completed, step back and, very slowly, release hands one at a time.

Stretches upper arms, chest, shoulders
Do not lead with head; tense or jut out neck; arch back; stick out buttocks

You will not get as much range of movement doing the pelvic wave in this stretch.

Experience how much pressure to put on your hands before doing full stretch.

UNDERARMS

1. Stand or sit with legs a hip-width apart, feet facing forward. Straighten legs but relax knees (don't lock them).

2. Stretch arms straight out to sides at shoulder level. Stretch torso two inches higher. Raise shoulders to ears. Slowly turn hands over, thumbs aiming toward your back, so that palms are facing ceiling. Try to aim thumbs toward ceiling.

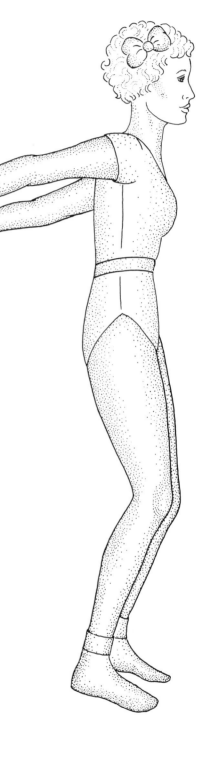

3. Holding head erect, tighten buttocks and curl up pelvis (pelvic wave). Slowly move arms behind you, as though you were trying to get backs of hands to touch; try to keep arms as high as possible. Hold for a count of 15 to 30. If you wish, after a count of 15, gently move hands back and forth toward each other no more than ¹⁄₁₆ inch, 5 to 10 times.

   NOTE: If you find this too difficult, try the exercises on pages 100–103.

It is more important to keep your arms straight than to keep them raised. However, concentrate on counteracting gravity by keeping your arms up.

Do not arch your back or stick your stomach out; let shoulders and head round forward.

Shoulders will naturally drop when taking arms to back or sides.

Stretches spine, neck, chest, and shoulders

Contracts buttocks, abdomen, front and inner thighs, underarms, between shoulder blades

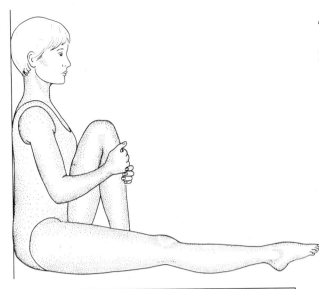

Stretches spine, neck, shoulders and chest

Do not *hold breath, arch back; slump or tense body*

SPINE

Beginner

1. Sit erect on floor, or against wall or door. Straighten right leg in front of you and bend left knee. Clasp hands and grasp left leg just below left knee.

2. Pull knee toward chest. Move forward with hips until you are sitting on "sit bones." Stretch torso and neck toward ceiling as high as possible (as though you were reaching two inches higher). Bring shoulders back as far as possible, flattening back against wall; pull chin in. Hold for a count of 20 to 30, stretching continuously.

3. Bend right knee and straighten left leg. Repeat stretch on other side.

Advanced

NOTE: If your foot doesn't reach the floor in the following exercise, you are not stretched enough. Do Stretch #12, page 57, instead.

Caution: If you have sciatica, do not straighten top leg out to side.

1. Lie on back with knees bent a hip-width apart and feet flat on floor. Arms are above head, elbows bent, backs of hands resting on floor.

2. Bend right leg and bring to chest in triple slow motion and straighten left leg, if possible. Roll right leg over to left side of body as far as possible, keeping elbows on floor all the time. Hold for a count of 60. If you wish, after a count of 30, move knee up and down no more than 1/16 inch, 5 to 10 times. When you are more stretched, your foot can touch the floor. In that position, move knee up and down. When you are even more stretched, your knee will touch the floor. From that position, either slide bent knee toward elbow or try to extend leg straight out to side.

3. In triple slow motion, bend knee and bring back to center; slowly lower right foot to floor. Bend left knee as in start position and repeat on other side.

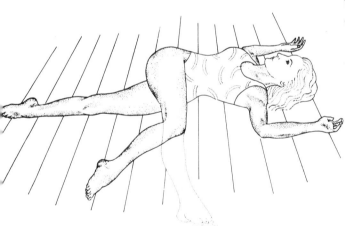

If you have a swayback, do pelvic wave to get more of a stretch.

Stretches chest, spine, hip flexors, neck, shoulders, outer thighs, buttocks; expands lungs

Do not *hold breath; crunch neck; bounce or jerk; tense body; arch back*

SPINAL TWIST

1. Sit on floor, with right leg stretched straight in front of you. Place left hand on floor behind you and rest weight on it. Bend left leg and cross over right leg, knee facing ceiling, resting foot on floor to outside of right knee. Stretch torso two inches higher.

2. Bend right elbow and press upper arm against outside of left knee. Slowly turn head toward left and gently try to look over left shoulder, while turning upper torso toward left hand. Hold for a count of 60. Or, if you wish, after a count of 15 to 30, move shoulder forward and back no more than ¹⁄₁₆ inch, 5 to 10 times.

3. Reverse and repeat on other side.

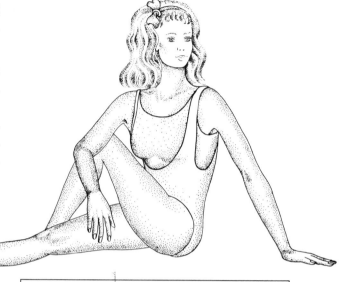

Stretches chest, spine, shoulders, neck, between shoulder blades; expands lungs

Do not *hold breath; tense body; arch back*

BRIDGING

1. Lie on back with knees bent, legs a hip-width apart, feet flat on floor. Arms are at your side, palms down on floor. Stretch neck and pull in chin.

2. Tighten buttocks and curl up pelvis (pelvic wave). Keep curling pelvis—it will go further than you think it will—until hips and buttocks automatically lift off floor. (It's all right if knees fall to side a little.) Maintain pelvic wave and raise torso until entire back is stretched straight. The more you do the pelvic wave, the more stretch you get in your spine. Your weight should be evenly distributed between your feet and your shoulders; feet should be light as feathers. Hold for a count of 60. If you wish, after a count of 15 to 30, curl back and forth no more than ¹⁄₁₆ inch, 5 to 10 times.

3. Slowly return torso to floor, one vertebra at a time. When you are flat on floor, release pelvic wave.

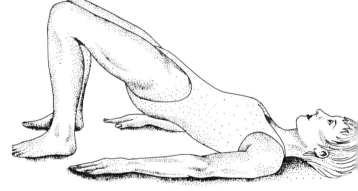

Stretches spine, neck; contracts buttocks, front and outer thigh muscles, hamstrings, abdominals, psoas (see page 170), vaginal muscles

Do not *rest solely on shoulders; arch back; crunch neck; grip feet; tense shoulders or neck*

WAIST

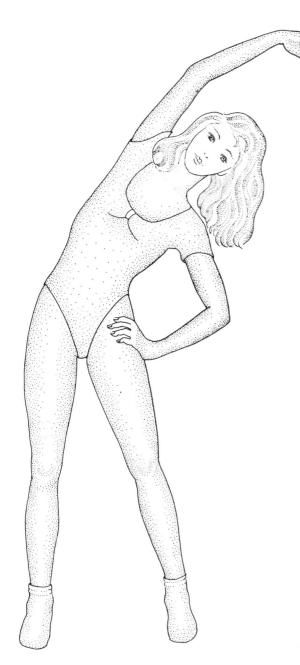

NOTE: For swayback or other discomfort, do not do this exercise. Instead, do "Waist, Stage III" (page 106).

1. Stand with legs a hip-width apart, knees slightly bent and relaxed, feet facing forward. Tighten buttocks and curl up pelvis (pelvic wave).

2. Place left hand just below left hip to support lower back, elbow pointed directly out to side. Raise right arm straight to ceiling, palm facing head, arm even with or slightly in front of right ear. Feel the stretch from your hip to the top of your fingers. Stretch as though you were reaching two inches higher. Start reaching directly over to left side, still stretching arm up as well as over. Imagine that upper body and arm are one unit and moving in same direction.

3. Move torso ¼ inch over to left side and back. Work up to 25 to 100 repetitions. Do not bounce or jerk. The smaller the motions, the greater the stretch and the more you will learn to be in control.

4. To reverse sides, reach forward with your right arm, really bend your knees deeply, and lean forward. Keeping left hand on hip, slowly move right arm (still reaching out) to other side.

5. To come out of position, bend knees more, place hands on hips or front thighs, tighten buttocks, and come up to standing position one vertebra at a time. Repeat on left side.

A good indication of how much you're stretching: You should feel your shorts or leotard riding up.

Stretches waist, between shoulder blades, entire spine, neck, arms

Do not arch back; tense shoulders; crunch neck; lock knees

FRONT THIGH (Quadriceps and Psoas)

Beginner

1. Stand facing wall, door, or other surface, and rest left hand on it for balance. Bend both knees.

2. Raise bent right leg, and with foot facing back grasp right foot with right hand. Tighten buttocks, curl up pelvis (pelvic wave). Pull leg to the back, feeling stretch in front thigh (quadriceps). Hold for a count of 15 to 30.

3. Gently return leg to floor and repeat on other side.

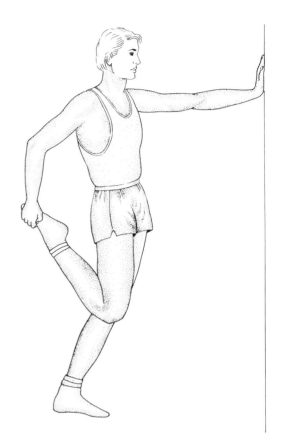

> *Stretches front thighs (quadriceps)*
>
> Do not *place heel on buttocks; arch back; lock knees; lead with head; pull leg to side*

Intermediate

1. Stand in front of a chair, facing away from it. Place left leg on chair (stand far enough away to feel a stretch in front of left thigh). Bend right knee, foot facing forward; tighten buttocks and curl up pelvis (pelvic wave).

2. Stand erect and pull chin in. (For balance, place hands on hips or some stable surface such as a wall.) Hold for a count of 60. If you wish, after a count of 15 to 30, tighten buttocks and curl up pelvis (pelvic wave); then try to curl up even more for a count of 5 to 10.

3. Return leg to floor and repeat on other side.

> *Stretches front thighs (quadriceps and psoas)*
>
> Do not *arch back*

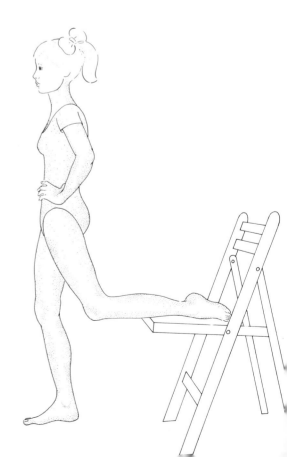

Advanced

1. Sit on heels, knees together or a hip-width apart. Place hands, palms down, on floor in back of body for support. Tighten buttocks and curl up pelvis (pelvic wave), still sitting on heels. Hold for a count of 30 to 60.

2. After you have done this enough to feel the

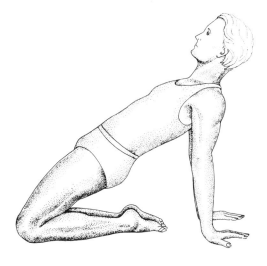

stretch in the front of your thighs, try to increase pelvic wave even more. Then lift buttocks off your heels as high as you can without arching lower back. Be sure to relax your neck. Hold for a count of 30 to 60.

3. Release buttocks and gently return to sitting on heels.

   NOTE: If you wish, place a folded towel or other light padding under knees and feet.

   For men: If you can't sit on heels, try sitting on toes, with heels off floor, or turning feet in and sitting on them.

PSOAS

When I was teaching the American Armed Forces in Europe, I was very surprised that so many of the competing athletes asked me if I had a particular stretch for the psoas muscle. I had assumed that anyone who used his or her body in competition would have realized that anytime you were lying down, with one leg straight on the floor and the other bent to the chest, the psoas was automatically being stretched. It occurred to me that, because of their intensive physical activity, these athletes would need a more effective stretch. When I demonstrated this, the only available surface was the floor of the competitive boxing ring; so I lay down under the ropes and hung my leg over the edge.

I know it's a nuisance to find the proper table for the length of your body, and then have to remove everything that has collected there, but this stretch is worth it.

1. Lie on your back on a stable surface (table, counter, etc.) with buttocks at edge.

2. Bring left knee to chest. Grasp leg in front, just below knee, with both hands. Pull knee in close enough to chest to get lower back as flat as possible on surface; pull chin in and relax shoulders. Let right leg dangle and allow gravity to do the stretching. Hold for a count of 15 to 30.

3. Bend dangling leg and bring to chest. Repeat on other side.

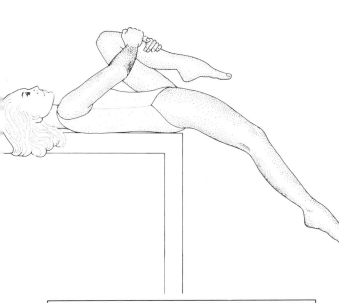

Stretches hip flexors, particularly psoas

Do not *arch back or neck*

INNER THIGHS

Beginner #1

1. Lie flat on back on floor, knees bent, feet on floor a hip-width apart. Bend elbows and place hands on abdomen. Slowly allow right leg to ease to floor on right side. Make sure to release all tension in hips and buttocks; gravity is doing the stretch.

2. Rest in this position for as long as you can, up to a count of 15 to 30. If you wish, after a count of 15, gently ease knee further to floor and back no more than 1/16 inch, 5 to 10 times.

3. Slowly return leg to starting position (you might want to assist it with your right hand). Repeat on other side.

NOTE: To avoid arching back, curl up pelvis (pelvic wave).

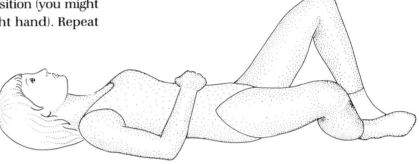

Beginner #2

1. Lie flat on back on floor, knees bent. Ease knees out to sides toward floor so that soles of feet are together. Relax legs. Bend elbows and place hands on abdomen.

2. Rest in this position for as long as you can, up to a count of 15 to 30; or, if you wish, after a count of 15, gently move knees no more than 1/16 inch toward floor and back, 10 times.

   NOTE: If you are swaybacked and feel your lower back is not flat enough on floor, tighten buttocks and curl up pelvis (pelvic wave) to decrease the hyperextension. Relax inner thighs.

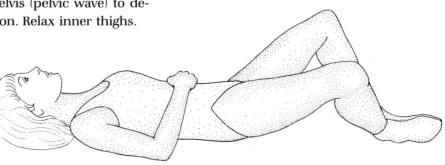

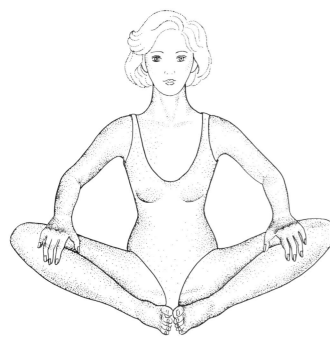

Intermediate #1

1. Sit on floor with back straight, chin pulled in, soles of feet together, knees out to side. Feet are a comfortable distance in front of body (the closer the heels are to midline, the greater the inner thigh stretch). Sit well forward on your "sit bones," or sit against a wall or door. (In the latter position, you will not be on your "sit bones" until you shift your hips forward.)

2. Very gently place hands on legs and lower them to floor. When you feel the stretch, hold for a count of 60. If you wish, after a count of 10 to 30, move legs up and down no more than $\frac{1}{16}$ inch, 5 to 10 times.

Intermediate #2

1. Sit on floor, knees bent, feet flat on floor, chin pulled in, and back of neck stretched as much as possible. Sit well forward on your "sit bones." Straighten right leg, on floor flex foot, and move leg out to right side as far as possible without forcing. Raise arms over head as high as possible to feel stretch through length of torso.

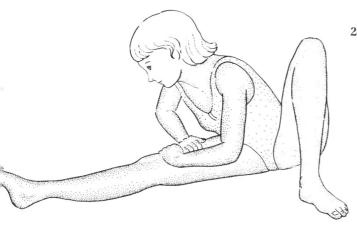

2. Slowly turn torso in direction of right foot. Stretch even higher to feel the stretch in your lower back. With the back as one unit, stretch torso forward from the hips over right leg as far as possible. (You may keep back straight or round upper back only.) Relax neck. Place hands next to each other, just above or below right knee and bend elbows out to side, to stretch between shoulder blades. Hold for a count of 60. If you wish, after holding for a count of 15 to 30, gently stretch torso forward and back $\frac{1}{16}$ inch, 5 to 10 times.

3. Reverse and repeat on other side.

NOTE: If you hold tension in your neck, make a conscious effort to let go of it. If you can't, bring head down when stretching forward over leg, neck and shoulders relaxed.

(continued)

INNER THIGHS, continued

Intermediate #3

1. Lie on back flat on floor, knees bent and feet on floor a hip-width apart.

2. Bring both knees, one at a time, up to chest and spread to shoulder-width. Place hands on inside of thighs above knees.

3. Gently ease knees with hands outward to sides of body. Hold for a count of 60, or, if you wish, after a count of 15 to 30, move them apart no more than 1/16 inch 5 to 10 times. If you are stretched enough, you can rest your elbows on floor.

4. Return to starting position. You may have to assist by placing hands on outside of knees and gently easing legs back to center.

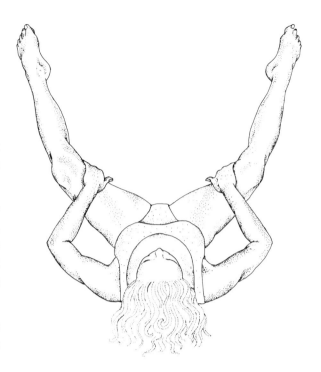

Advanced #1

1. Lie on back flat on floor, knees bent and feet on floor a hip-width apart.

2. Bring both knees, one at a time, up to chest and spread to shoulder-width. Place hands on inside of thighs above knees.

3. Gently ease knees with hands outward to side of body. Hold for a count of 60; if you wish, after a count of 15 to 30, move them apart no more than 1/16 inch, 5 to 10 times. If you are stretched enough, you can rest elbows on floor.

4. With hands on inside of thighs just above knees, straighten legs upward; then stretch

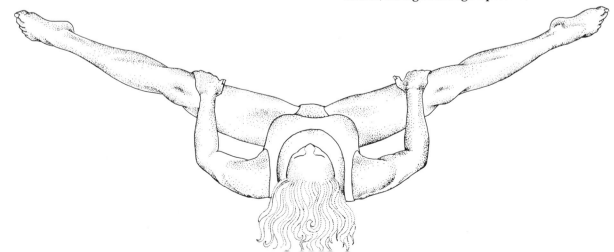

open as far as possible. Hold for a count of 10 to 60; if you wish, after a count of 15, gently move legs no more than ¹⁄₁₆ inch farther apart, 5 to 10 times.

5. Bend knees, bringing them close to body; place hands on outside of thighs just above knees and slowly return legs to center and then, one at a time, to floor.

   Caution: If you have sciatica, do not straighten legs completely.

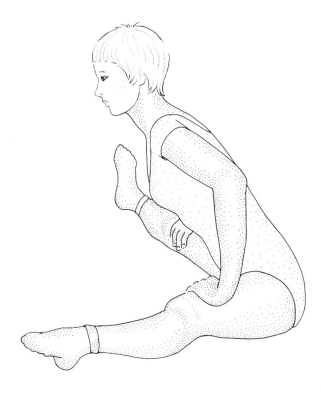

NOTE: Round only upper back, not lower. This will protect your lower back. Relax neck and shoulders.

Inner Thighs Advanced #2

1. Sit erect on floor with legs as straight as possible, out to the sides. (You can move your legs farther out by grasping each one on the inside thigh and lifting one leg at a time until you are in a more stretched position.) Keep back of neck stretched and chin pulled in. Place hands, palms down, behind you, next to buttocks, and shift weight forward onto "sit bones."

2. Place hands above knees or straight out in front, resting on floor. Bend torso forward at hips. Hold for a count of 15 to 30; work up to a count of 60. If you wish, after a count of 30, gently stretch torso forward and back ¹⁄₁₆ inch, 5 to 10 times; keep lower back straight.

3. Place hands on floor and walk them back. Round your upper back and very slowly return to sitting erect, one vertebra at a time.

4. Let right hand rest on right leg anywhere except knee. Stretch left arm straight up. Turn torso toward right leg, nose aiming at right foot and then over, as though you were going to touch foot with your hand. When you feel the pull, place hands above or below right knee and bend elbows out to side. (You can also place your palms on floor on either side of leg.) Hold for a count of 60. If you wish, after holding for a count of 30, stretch torso forward and back ¹⁄₁₆ inch, 5 to 10 times.

5. Walk hands back as you return to sitting erect one vertebra at a time. Repeat on other side.

CALVES/ACHILLES

#1

1. Sit erect on floor, with legs straight in front of you a hip-width apart. Bend right knee to point where heel is in line with left leg anywhere between knee and ankle (the closer to the knee, the greater the stretch).

2. Shift forward with hips to sit on "sit bones." Bend from the hips, stretch arms, and grasp toes of right foot with both hands. Flex foot toward chest.

3. Keeping lower back straight, round upper back. Try to gently pull toes toward chest with hands, at the same time pulling torso away from foot. Hold for a count of 15 to 30. If you wish, after holding for a count of 15, pull flexed foot forward even more, no more than 1/16 inch, 5 to 10 times.

4. Repeat on other side.

Stretches calves, Achilles tendon, spine, neck, between shoulder blades (if elbows are out); contracts arm muscles

Do not arch back; slump; round lower back; tense neck; hunch shoulders

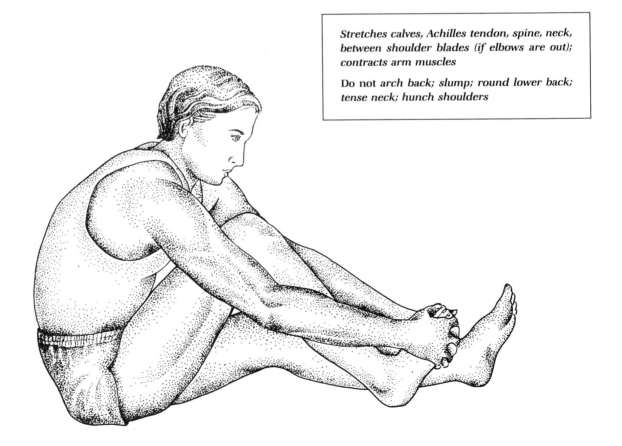

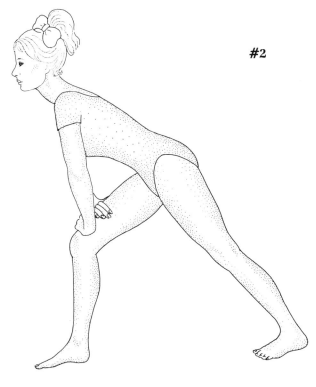

#2

1. Stand with legs a hip-width apart. Move left leg about 18 inches directly to the back and bend right knee. Toes of both feet are pointing forward; head is relaxed and eyes are facing front.

2. Bend from hips and place both hands on front thigh, elbows out to side. Tighten buttocks and curl up pelvis (pelvic wave), and push left heel into floor. Hold for a count of 15 to 30. If you wish, after a count of 30, bend right knee more and move forward and back no more than $\frac{1}{16}$ inch, 5 to 10 times.

3. Repeat on other leg.

   NOTE: This exercise can be done with arms outstretched with hands resting on a wall or door. The important point is to feel the stretch in the back calf.

> *Stretches calves, Achilles tendon, spine, hamstrings, inner thighs, neck*
>
> Do not *lead with head; arch back; hunch shoulders; lock knees*

#3

1. Stand facing a wall or counter, at straight arm's length. Keeping arms a shoulder-width apart at a comfortable height, place hands against wall. Step back 12 inches, being careful not to lock elbows. Keep feet together, facing front.

2. Raise left foot in front of you no higher than level of right knee. Press right heel into floor hard. Tighten buttocks and curl up pelvis (pelvic wave), relax right knee, gently lean torso forward. (Both legs should be totally relaxed.) Hold for a count of 60. If you wish, after a count of 15 to 30, gently move torso forward and back no more than $\frac{1}{16}$ inch, 5 to 10 times.

3. Lower left leg to floor and repeat on other side.

> *Stretches calves, Achilles tendons, hamstrings, inner thighs, and spine*
>
> Do not arch back; stick out stomach; lock knees.

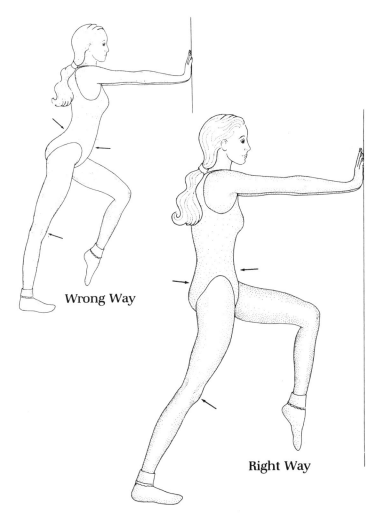

Wrong Way

Right Way

HAMSTRINGS

NOTE: Tight hamstrings often aggravate lower back problems. For this reason, it is very important to stretch hamstrings; if they are not stretched, you cannot straighten legs completely. Many people have tight hamstrings (it's one of the most difficult muscles to stretch and keep stretched). I have not labeled these exercises in stages; the degree of your flexibility will determine how far you can go. In many of the following stretches, I indicate a progression toward increased flexibility. For some, total flexibility will not be possible; for others, practice will yield greater flexibility. *Patience* and *relaxation* are the key words. Under no circumstances should you force the stretch or compare your flexibility with others. When you feel you're really stretched, you can flex foot toward body. This will stretch calf as well.

HAMSTRINGS #1

1. Sit on floor with back straight, legs hip-width apart, right leg straight out in front and left leg bent, foot in line with right knee; left hand is under left thigh. Pull chin in.

2. Shift hips forward to sit on your "sit bones." Slowly, bend from the hips, lower back straight, reaching right arm over right foot. Hold for a count of 60. If you wish, after count of 30, *slowly* move torso forward and back no more than ¹⁄₁₆ inch, 10 to 20 times.

3. Bend right leg, straighten left and repeat on other side.

   NOTE: If you flex foot on straightened leg, the calf gets a good stretch.

#2

1. Sit erect on floor or against wall or door. Straighten left leg in front of you; bend right knee and rest heel on left thigh. Grasp back of right leg above knee with right hand and grasp under the ankle with left hand.

2. Gently bring leg up toward the chest as close as possible, without forcing. Hold for a count of 60. If you wish, after a count of 30, gently pull bent leg forward and back no more than ¹⁄₁₆ inch, 10 to 20 times.

3. Slowly return bent leg to floor and repeat on other side.

   NOTE: This exercise also stretches buttocks muscles. It can also be done in a chair.

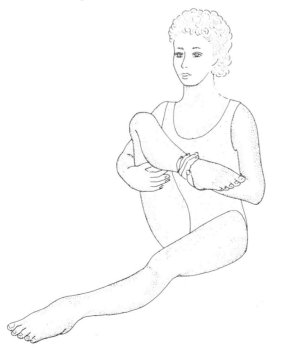

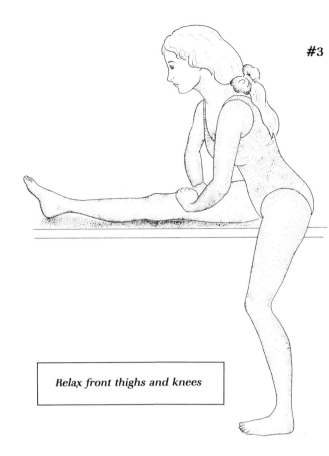

#3

Relax front thighs and knees

Caution: Do not do the following stretch if you have sciatica; instead, do the hamstring stretch on page 127.

1. Stand alongside counter or table (hip height or lower) and bend both knees. Raise right leg and rest buttocks and leg on surface. Left foot should be facing forward.

2. Raise arms over head and stretch torso toward ceiling as high as possible (as though you were two inches taller). Bend forward from hips, keeping lower back straight, to the point where you feel a stretch in your hamstring. Place both hands on right thigh, elbows out to side, and hold for a count of 60. If you wish, stretch a little further after a count of 30 and hold again before releasing; or move your torso forward and back no more than ¹/₁₆ inch, 10 to 20 times.

3. Slowly bend right leg and return to floor, turn around, and repeat on other side.

#4

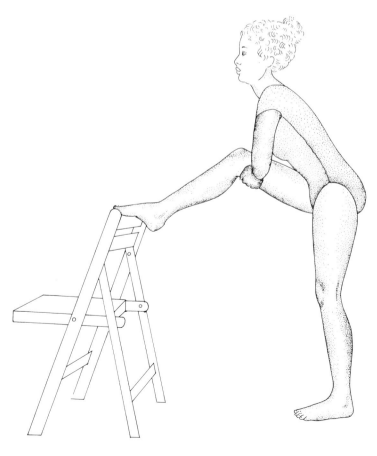

Caution: Do not do the following stretch if you have sciatica; instead, do the hamstring stretch on page 127.

1. Stand facing table, counter, or sturdy chair, back straight and chin pulled in. Bend right knee, raise right leg, and place arch or ball of foot on edge of surface. Try to keep standing, leg facing front; do not lock knee.

2. Stretch torso toward ceiling, as though you were reaching two inches higher. Still stretching, bend from the hips over right leg. Clasp hands behind right thigh, or rest on front of thigh, not knees. Keep elbows out to sides. Hold for a count of 60. If you wish, after a count of 30, move body forward and back no more than ¹/₁₆ inch, 10 to 20 times.

3. Slowly return right leg to floor and repeat on other side.

NOTE: You can round the top of your back to increase the stretch in the upper back.

(continued)

HAMSTRINGS, *continued*

#5

1. Stand erect in front of an object on the floor (book, box, etc.) that is at least 12 inches high. Legs are a hip-width apart. Bend both knees, tighten buttocks, and curl up pelvis (pelvic wave). Bend from the hips, keeping back straight or rounding upper back and keeping lower back straight.

2. Place palms on object and slowly begin to straighten left leg until you feel a gentle stretch in hamstring. Hold for a count of 60. Bend left knee, straighten right leg, and repeat on other side. When you are really stretched, you can do this stretch with both legs at the same time, knees relaxed.

3. When you have completed this stretch, bend knees, do pelvic wave, and slowly return to standing position, one vertebra at a time.

   NOTE: The object you rest on can be any height, but the higher it is, the less stretch you will get. As you increase your flexibility, you can reduce the height of the object until you are doing this stretch with both palms on the floor.

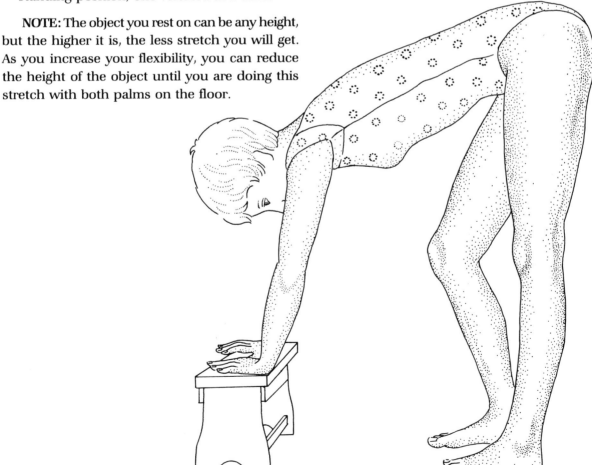

NECK

Caution: Do the neck stretches only when you have time to fully concentrate on them and can do them in triple slow motion. People with swaybacks (this is one of my problems) should bend knees more to feel how even they can straighten the lower back.

All these stretches may also be done while sitting in a chair or on the floor, whichever feels better for your lower back.

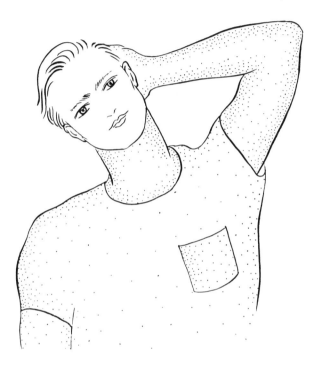

Beginner

1. Stand erect with legs a hip-width apart, knees slightly bent. Tighten buttocks and curl up pelvis (pelvic wave). Relax shoulders; do not make the common mistake of tensing them and holding them under the ears.

2. Stretch neck and, keeping shoulders relaxed and down, slowly lower head to the right, so that your right ear is as close as possible to your right shoulder, nose pointing straight ahead.

3. Place left hand on left side of head. Very gently press head toward your right shoulder. Hold for a count of 5.

4. Slowly return head to center. Stretch neck up toward ceiling, chin pulled in (not down). Repeat on other side.

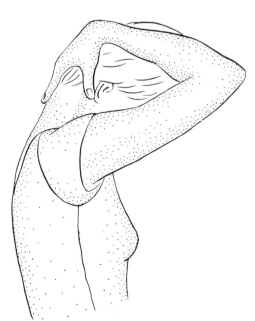

Advanced

1. Stand with knees slightly bent, legs a hip-width apart. Tighten buttocks and curl up pelvis (pelvic wave). Relax shoulders.

2. Stretch neck up, pull chin in. Place one hand, fingers pointing downward, on base of skull. While still stretching up, gently press head down with hand until nose is aimed toward floor. Hold for a count of 5.

3. Release pressure of hand, but keep it there, and in triple slow motion return head to upright position.

   NOTE: The position of the head and neck in this exercise is the same as shown on page 112 for the abdominal exercises and is excellent practice for these.

BUTTOCKS

1

1. Sit on floor with legs crossed (Indian style) comfortably in front of you (about 8 to 10 inches), right leg in front, back straight, arms resting at sides.

2. Cross right leg over bent left knee, which is even with midline of body, and rest right foot on floor, toes facing forward, in front of left knee.

3. Bend left arm and lean weight over to left side. Stretch right arm forward straight on the floor as far as possible. Very gently, try to press right buttock toward floor. (Bottom of foot will raise up.) Hold for a count of 30 to 60.

4. Reverse and repeat on other side.

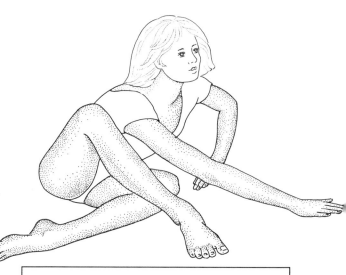

Stretches buttocks, spine, outer thighs

BUTTOCKS

2

1. Sit on floor with legs crossed comfortably in front of you (right leg in front), spine straight, arms resting on legs.

2. Sit on "sit bones." Place both hands on floor in front of you and walk hands forward, one at a time, as far as possible without forcing. Hold for a count of 10 to 20. If you wish, after a count of 10, move torso very gently forward and back no more than ¹⁄₁₆ an inch, 5 to 10 times. Adjust position of legs if you feel discomfort in hip joints.

3. Walk hands over toward left foot; bend torso forward over left foot. Hold for a count of 30 to 60. If you wish, after a count of 30, move torso very gently forward and back over foot no more than ¹⁄₁₆ inch, 5 to 10 times.

4. Switch legs so that left leg is in front and walk hands toward right foot. Bend torso over right foot and repeat movements in step 3.

5. Walk hands to center and return to sitting position, one vertebra at a time.

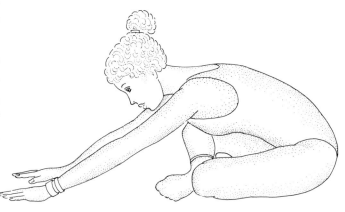

Stretches buttocks, spine, and outer thighs

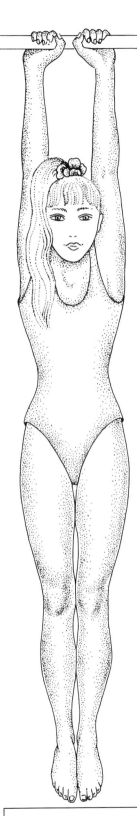

Stretches muscles of arms, shoulders and torso;

strengthens hands and wrists

Do relax

HANGING

Equipment: Do not attempt any hanging exercises unless you have the proper equipment. You will need a chinning bar, sold in sporting goods stores, which fits into brackets permanently attached to a door frame (the bar can be removed; the brackets are screwed in). A stool may be needed if the bar is too high to reach without standing on toes; suction bars without supports are not safe enough. You may also try this stretch on sturdy bars in your gym or playground.

Precautionary measures: If you have a shoulder injury or painful condition, do not do this stretch. When hanging, your feet should never be more than 2 to 3 inches from the floor.

NOTE: The height of the bar does not matter; you will get the stretch at any height, by kneeling, sitting, or hanging. Do not be concerned about how long you can hold the stretch; if you can hang only for a count of 1—fine. When I started doing this, I could only reach a very fast count of 5 because my wrists were so weak. Now I can almost fall asleep while hanging! And my body feels 4 inches taller. You will be amazed that in no time at all your wrists will become so strong that you will be able to count up to 20, 30, or more. Many people at first have a fear of losing their grip and will tend to tense the body, especially the lower back, to help them hold on. This doesn't help at all; on the contrary, it's defeating the purpose and exhausting the body. No matter how long you hang, you should maintain control at all times so that you can get on and off the stool slowly, safely, and gracefully. Once you gain confidence, it feels wonderful!

Hanging Straight

1. Place a sturdy stool on floor, slightly in front of bar. Stand on stool and curl hands around bar, fingers facing forward. Slowly take one foot off stool and let leg stretch down. Then slowly take the other foot off so that you are hanging free.

2. Hold for as long as you can. Try to hang as straight as possible. *Do not arch back.* Relax and feel as though entire body is going to sink into floor. This is a perfect time to realize how much you are tensing your lower back. Concentrate on releasing it. Keep in mind that it has nothing to do with preventing you from falling.

3. Slowly put one foot back on the stool; repeat with other foot.

Advanced: As you progress, you can begin to do the pelvic wave while hanging for a greater stretch.

Sitting: If you hang your bar lower, you can either sit on the floor or on a stool to reach up. Make sure your arms are straight and bar is high enough to feel the stretch in your spine.

CAT STRETCH

NOTE: If you are swaybacked, you must maintain the pelvic wave throughout this entire stretch, until you're resting on your heels, to prevent arching your back (hyperextension).

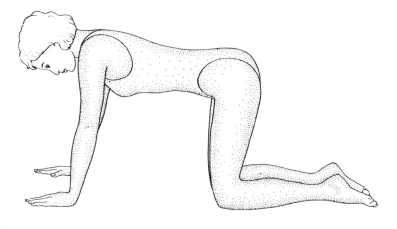

1. With carpet, pad or folded towel to protect your knees, kneel on floor on all fours, back straight, knees hip-width apart or together, hands a shoulder-width apart.

2. Slowly round back as much as possible, allowing head to gently hang down. Hold for count of 5.

3. Slowly return to original position. Repeat 5 times. Round back more each time; you can stretch it more than you think.

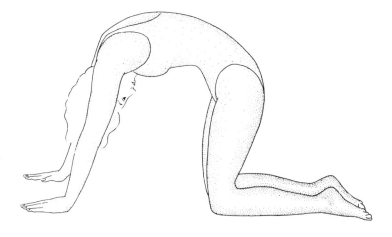

4. Complete this stretch by going in to the knee-chest stretch: From the original position, slowly stretch buttocks toward heels and feel upper body stretch forward on floor. Keep arms straight out on floor. Once you are on your heels, you can walk hands farther forward to increase upper body stretch. Relax neck; if possible rest forehead on floor. Hold for count of 5 or as long as you feel like. Relax; really concentrate on feeling your body melt into the floor.

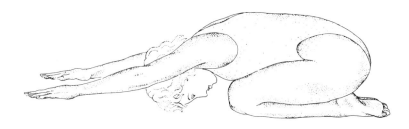

Stretches: spine, neck, shoulders, arms; counteracts round shoulders

Do relax; take advantage of lying down to let your body feel like wax melting onto the floor

3.

Minnie Mouse's Shoes and Other Foot Travesties

What have the feet got to do with the back? Quite a lot. Yet few of us realize how much our feet affect our backs and vice versa.

Feet are extremely complex in structure. They have to be; they were designed to bear as much as three times your body weight each time you walk—and you take about eight thousand steps every day. Imagine the impact of that weight on your poor feet. And imagine the impact of that weight on your back. The way the body weight is balanced on the feet is another key factor. While standing, an average body weighing anywhere from 125 to 200 pounds balances on a base that is less than one square foot; and then this extremely narrow base is reduced by half in the act of walking, because the weight shifts each time to only one foot, not both. Considering these dynamics, it's easy for imbalances to occur. Anything that causes an imbalance—from osteoarthritis to poor posture—can affect the feet and actually cause abnormal foot function and structure. The model of good alignment depends on distribution of body weight on the bones of the feet. Most of us cannot measure up to that standard. Even such problems as calluses and bunions can be the result of poor spinal alignment; calluses are nature's way of protecting bony prominences (bunions) and grow on areas where you place the most pressure. In most instances, when there are calluses on the bottom of a foot, it's a sure sign that something is out of alignment—either in the foot, leg, knee, or back. If you ever had a thick callus shaved down, did you notice that it affected your balance for the first day or so?

There is a distinct relationship between the spinal vertebrae and the feet: The nerves radiating from the area between the fifth lumbar vertebra (the one in the lower back that is so vulnerable) and the sacrum (see pages 170–171) activate movement of the feet. So intertwined is the connection between the feet and the back that it is often difficult to see what is affecting what. Sometimes the answer only comes from your own experimentation or consulting either a podiatrist or back specialist.

THE LAST PHASE IN THE TORTURE OF WOMEN

The feet have enemies. What first comes to mind are shoes.

Although my feet ached when I spent all those years wearing rubber thongs and bearing the weight of my rucksack, I never went into "screaming" lower back spasm until I began wearing Western-style shoes. I am at war with the shoe industry. I'm really angry that they think that women wear only one size shoe. When I was growing up, you could get sizes up to an E width. Today, everything is called "medium." Yet feet tend to get wider with age. If you love to see people tortured, sit in a store where women are trying on shoes—especially high heels—and watch their expressions. You can see exactly when it gets painful. But women will not admit it, because they want their feet to look smaller and daintier, and the manufacturers capitalize on this.

Men don't have this problem, because the manufacturers actually makes shoes to fit them. Isn't it amusing that the most fashionable shoes for women are designed by men who never walked in anything like them? In the French court a few hundred years ago, it was the fashion for men to wear heels, and guess what—one of the royal Louis (I forget who) was complaining about his aching back! Nowadays, how often do you hear salesmen or men saying at a cocktail party, "Oh, my shoes are killing me! I just have to sit down." Never! It's always women—and not only women in heels.

Most shoes give no support, no cushion on the ball of the foot or the heel. I wear a size 5 shoe, but I have to buy a 7 for the width, and then, naturally, it slips off the back of my foot. So I have to cram all sorts of pads and heel guards to take even one step. My shoes are so big and clumsy, I look like Minnie Mouse. But I can't help it because there must be enough space in the front for the toes to wiggle and be separated. Is that a dream today?

Women get curled-up toes, bunions (unsightly bone deformities), and blisters all from ill-fitting shoes. If women were more concerned with their health and less with their distorted idea of beauty, they would realize that an unblemished foot (even if it's wide) is a lot prettier and more feminine, and certainly healthier, than one with all those self-inflicted "deformities."

Now let's talk about high heels. If you want a dramatic example of how feet can affect your back, put on a pair of high heels, walk around for a while, and notice how your lower back feels. I'm sure it hurts many of you. That's because you're shifting more weight to the balls of your feet, which causes your pelvis to be thrust forward, your behind to stick out, your back to arch, and your lower back

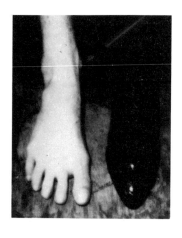

Foot shoe: Every foot is supposed to fit into a shoe that is so narrow it looks like a Barbie doll's. How is it physically, mentally, and emotionally possible to fit *this* size 5 wide foot into *this* 6½ medium shoe?

muscles to contract. It's totally logical that the broader the base, the better the weight can be balanced. When you wear high heels, most of the weight is moved to the front of the shoe, which is usually the narrowest part, especially those fashionable lethal pointed toes. The higher the heel, the less stable your ankle joint. Therefore, heels can cause you to be more prone to spraining your ankles.

When I went to parties and wanted to wear heels, I'd leave the house in ballet slippers. The reason was that not only are ballet slippers so comfortable, but they are also small and will fit easily into a handbag. I'd carry my heels in a beautiful little cotton bag, and right before I'd get to the party I'd put them on and no one was the wiser. Then I'd join the party, automatically head for a sofa or a chair, and sit there the entire time, appearing like Poor Pitiful Pearl, all by myself.

After a while I stopped going to parties because by wearing heels for even as short a distance as the front door to the couch, the next morning one hip would be higher than the other.

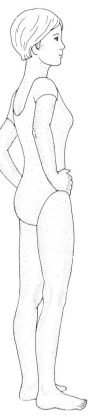

My fantasy is to be buried in a short white Belgian lace dress, wearing leg makeup (to hide my freckles) and a beautiful pair of red high heels. I think that's the only time I'll ever be able to wear heels comfortably!

What if you can't bear to give up your lovely high heels altogether? I know I can't. If you could find shoes that were wide in the front, you could probably handle a one-inch heel with no difficulty at all. The way I manage to walk at all in high heels is to continually do the pelvic wave (tighten buttocks, curl up pelvis—see pages 88–90). A good idea is to switch off; if you wear high heels at night, change to comfortable lower ones the next day. But be careful not to vary heights too drastically because it will put too much stress on the back. Some women can't wear shoes that are altogether flat, because they're so used to wearing heels that the Achilles tendon has been shortened.

I like to go barefoot as often as possible. However, I've been told by some podiatrists that you must be careful about the surfaces you walk on. Walking barefoot on a hard surface is jarring and may eventually cause back pain. Also, if you are not aligned and do not walk evenly, walking barefoot may be even worse than wearing shoes. (Even in societies where walking barefoot is the norm, people get bunions and calluses.)

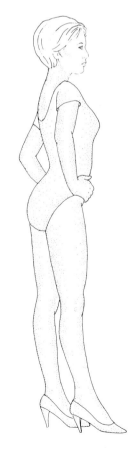

The ideal shoes are soft, cushioned, low, and wide enough to accommodate the front of your foot comfortably, with good support, flexibility and shock absorbency. In fact, in a study of back sufferers, a large percentage of the people who wore lightweight flexible-sole shoes fitted with shock-absorbing cushions experienced rapid back pain relief. So when it comes to protecting the back, the issue is as much the entire fit and cushioning of the shoe as it is the height of the heel. These kinds of shoes will help keep you balanced, improve your posture, relieve and prevent back pain. And don't forget toenails: Any shoe will fit better if toenails are properly clipped.

There is no lack of helpers for the feet, ranging from bunion regulators (a sort of sling to cushion bunions and straighten toes) to metatarsal cradles to heel cups to foot-fixer machines to electric massagers. The one I find most important for back health is a small shoe insert called an orthotic. Specially prescribed and fitted by a foot or back specialist, orthotics strengthen certain muscles and relax others. They can help redistribute your weight, equalize the length of your legs, and compensate for certain abnormalities, such as flattened arches (flat feet.) I am a champion of orthotics due to the fact that my feet were twisted at birth, and this appliance became a necessity for me as an adult. They have definitely helped my back, and all my students who wore them said they were a gift from heaven.

It's a good idea to keep your feet and toes flexible. Foot and leg exercises can be done while watching television, bathing, getting dressed, sitting, or standing. Many of the exercises in Three Stages of Callanetics, particularly the pelvic wave and pelvic rotations (pages 88–93 and 132–135) are excellent for the feet in relation to the back. In addition, you can do the following:
- With your hands, twist feet, pull toes, bend toes forward and backward.
- Wiggle your toes often.
- Stretch your toes apart, trying to separate them.
- Walk barefoot on soft sand.
- Massage feet, particularly the arch and metatarsals; try to separate the bones.
- Elevate your feet by lying on your back and resting them against a wall. This is an excellent way to relax tired legs and feet. Or take a warm foot bath.
- Do an Achilles stretch (see stretches for calves pages 38–39).

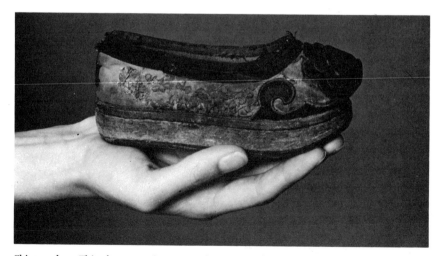

Chinese shoe: This shoe was given to me by my grandmother as a memento of her trip to China in 1912. It barely fills my palm. The binding of their feet was so brutal that most Chinese women had to be carried on palanquins. I was told that during the Second World War, when the Chinese had to evacuate a place in a hurry, the women were left behind because they had such difficulty walking. Imagine—it took four men to carry one female, and these men were running for their lives from the invading Japanese! By the way, this tortuous binding caused the foot to be "bowed"—very similar to the position in a high heel!

4.

Stretches for a Bad Back

The following gentle motions should be practiced daily to help alleviate back pain and prevent back problems. Stiffness occurs mostly when you're sleeping; in order to loosen your joints, these are effective motions to do in bed before getting up or just upon arising. It's preferable to do them on a firm surface. They can also serve as your warm-ups before starting any other gentle exercises. If you prefer, they can be done before going to bed to ease any discomfort or tension built up during the day and to relax you, making sleep more comfortable.

To achieve a healthy back you must maintain, throughout all your daily activities, correct posture, strength, and flexibility. By doing these stretching and strengthening exercises regularly, you will be taking an important first step toward this goal. As with any body movement, the more you practice, the more proficient you will become; and soon your body will automatically function in the best way to protect your back.

I have adapted these standard exercises and put them in a particular sequence so that you will be able to move through the entire program with ease. In addition, they start with elementary motions (good for even the most severe problems) and progress, while gradually loosening you up, into areas that are more difficult at first to stretch. This gives you an opportunity to exercise according to your own pace and ability. The final stretch is designed to totally relax you.

Do not think of these as mechanical motions. For people in pain, they are truly pleasurable, and you will actually look forward to doing them. Instead of being at the mercy of your condition, there is great satisfaction in knowing that *you* can be in control of your own healing process. This gives you a wonderful opportunity to bring your consciousness to the areas that need the most help. Your imagination can help you to stroke, caress, and soothe the pain away. (Some people even play war games: the good armies [comfort] against the bad armies [pain].) Naturally, while all this is happening, you will be deriving physical benefits from the motions as well.

All of the following exercises are done lying down. You may do them on the floor, a bed, or any other firm surface. There is an art to lying on the floor. For most people the tendency is to lie with the back arched. To prevent this, bend your knees, feet on the floor, and wiggle your body around until you are in a position where your lower back is melting into the floor. Do not forcefully tighten your abdominals (no matter what you've heard)—they automatically contract and need no extra assistance from you. When you deliberately tighten them, you may also have a tendency to tighten your lower back, preventing it from melting into the floor. And if your lower back is not totally relaxed into the floor, your pelvis cannot curl up enough for you to get the maximum stretch you need for the lower back— which is the purpose of these motions. People with swaybacks must be particularly conscious of letting the lower back melt into the floor and should train themselves to acquire that sensation.

Some people may find the following exercises more comfortable if they use a small folded towel or pillow placed under the sacrum (right above the tailbone) and/or under the neck.

NOTE: In all these exercises, the starting position is the same. When you have completed an exercise, gently return to the starting position, but never straighten your legs unless specified. <u>All movements should be done in triple slow motion.</u>

Don't be concerned about the "correct" way to breathe at this point; just breathe naturally.

Getting down, the right way

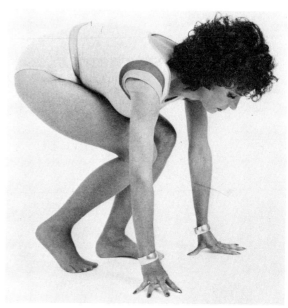

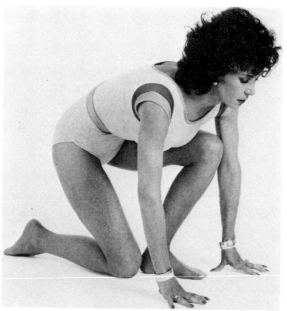

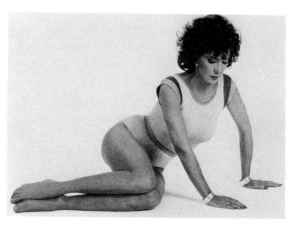

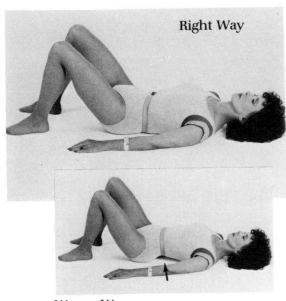

Right Way

Wrong Way

BACK STRETCH #1

1. Lie on floor, knees bent, feet on floor a hip-width apart, 1 to 1½ feet from buttocks. Arms are straight and resting on floor next to body. Stretch muscles at back of neck, as though you were going to flatten it on floor; then relax it. (I find it easy to do this if I position my head with my hands.) Keep jaw relaxed.

2. Press small of back into floor by tightening buttocks muscles.

3. Gently curl up pelvis in direction of navel (pelvic wave). Hold for a count of 5; release slowly back to floor to a count of 5. Repeat 5 times in slow motion. Each time you repeat, allow pelvis to curl up toward navel even more.

BACK STRETCH #2

1. Lie on floor, knees bent, feet on floor a hip-width apart, 1 to 1½ feet from buttocks. Arms are straight and resting on floor next to body. Stretch muscles at back of neck, as though you were going to flatten it on floor; then relax it.

2. Raise right knee toward chest. Place hands in front of leg below knee or in back of thigh and gently hug knee to chest. Hold for a count of 5.

3. Lower leg very slowly. Repeat motion with left leg. Do 5 sets.

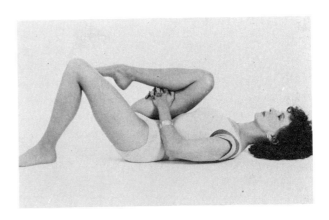

BACK STRETCH #3

1. Lie on floor, knees bent, feet on floor a hip-width apart, 1 to 1½ feet from buttocks. Arms are straight and resting on floor next to body. Stretch muscles at back of neck, as though you were going to flatten it on floor; then relax it.

2. Raise both knees, one at a time, toward chest at shoulder-width. Place hands in front of legs below knees or hold back of thighs and gently hug knees to chest. Hold for a count of 5. Pull just enough to feel that lower back is stretching and tailbone is coming off floor. Hold for count of 5.

3. Slowly lower legs, one at a time, to floor, keeping knees bent.

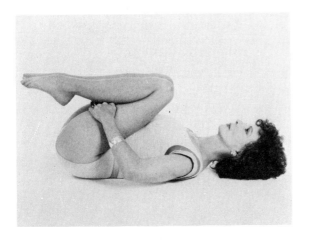

BACK STRETCH #4

1. Lie on floor, knees bent, feet on floor a hip-width apart, 1 to 1½ feet from buttocks. Arms are above head, elbows bent, backs of hands resting on floor. Stretch muscles at back of neck, as though you were going to flatten it on floor; then relax it.

2. Bring legs up to chest one at a time. Gently roll legs, one at a time, over to left side. Keep shoulders on floor if you can. Rest in this position for a count of 5 to 10.

3. Bring legs back, one at a time, to center. Gently repeat to left side.

4. Return legs to starting position, one at a time, keeping knees bent.

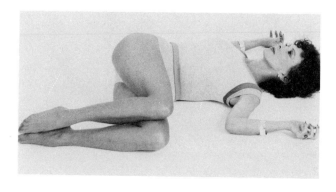

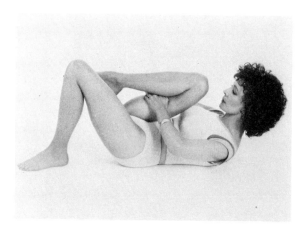

BACK STRETCH #6

1. Lie on floor, knees bent, feet on floor a hip-width apart, 1 to 1½ feet from buttocks. Arms are straight and resting on floor next to body. Stretch muscles at back of neck, as though you were going to flatten it on floor; then relax it.

2. Rest left foot on right thigh. Place hands behind head (only to support weight of head), elbows out. Slowly raise upper body, bringing right elbow and left knee toward each other. Hold for a count of 5. Slowly lower upper body.

3. Repeat on other side. Work up to 5 sets.

BACK STRETCH #5

1. Lie on floor, knees bent, feet on floor a hip-width apart, 1 to 1½ feet from buttocks. Arms are straight and resting on floor next to body. Stretch muscles at back of neck, as though you were going to flatten it on floor; then relax it.

2. Raise right knee to chest and clasp with both hands just under back of thigh. With elbows out to side, gently bring forehead toward knee. (Objective is not to have forehead touch knee, merely to aim toward it.) Hold for count of 5.

3. Gently lower head, then leg, still keeping knee bent. Do 5 sets. Repeat on other side. Hold for count of 5. Do 5 sets.

NOTE: In Stretches #5 and #6, if you feel discomfort in your neck, it is probably due to tension. Concentrate on relaxing, and this should improve as you continue to do the stretches. If it does not improve, you might want to consult a health professional.

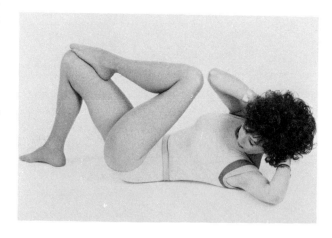

BACK STRETCH #7

Caution: If you have sciatica, check with your doctor before doing this exercise.

1. Lie on floor, knees bent, feet on floor a hip-width apart, 1 to 1½ feet from buttocks. Arms are straight and resting on floor next to body. Stretch muscles at back of neck, as though you were going to flatten it on floor; then relax it.

2. Place hands behind head. Bring right leg up, straightening it toward ceiling, as much as you can, until you feel a stretch in back of the legs. (If your hamstrings are tight, do not force your leg to straighten totally.) Flex foot by pointing toes toward nose; then point toes toward ceiling. Flex and point 5 times.

3. Rotate foot in small circles, moving only from the ankle, to a count of 5.

4. Gently bend knee and return leg to starting position. Repeat on other side.

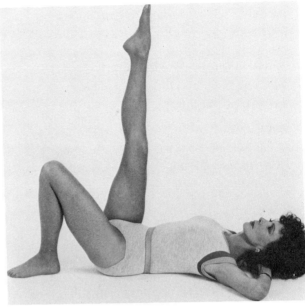

NOTE: When you feel stretched enough, grasp leg behind your calf (or, if you can't reach, behind your thigh) and with elbows out, gently pull leg toward face. Keep foot relaxed; do not jerk. Hold for count of 5 to 30. With consistent practice you will eventually be able to do this with ease.

BACK STRETCH #8

1. Lie on floor, knees bent, feet on floor a hip-width apart, 1 to 1½ feet from buttocks. Arms are straight and resting on floor next to body. Stretch muscles at back of neck, as though you were going to flatten it on floor; then relax it.

2. Bring both knees, one at a time, up to chest and spread to shoulder-width. Place palms on inside of legs.

3. With hands, gently move knees outward to sides of body as far as you can without forcing. Hold for a count of 5 to 60. If you are stretched enough, you can rest your elbows on the floor.

4. Still holding legs, return to starting position. Gently ease legs back to center and down, one at a time. (You might have to assist legs by placing hands on outside of knees.)

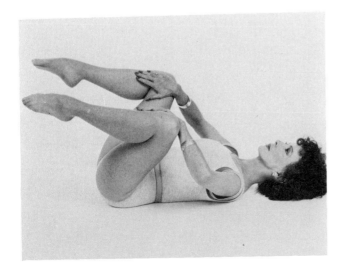

BACK STRETCH #9

1. Lie on floor, knees bent, feet on floor a hip-width apart, 1 to 1½ feet from buttocks. Arms are straight and resting on floor next to body. Stretch muscles at back of neck, as though you were going to flatten it on floor; then relax it.

2. Bring both knees up to chest, one at a time, and spread to shoulder-width. Grasp inside of legs well below knees.

3. Gently curl up pelvis in direction of navel, enough so that tailbone comes 1 inch off floor. Hold for a count of 5. Release pelvis slowly back to floor to a count of 5. Repeat 5 times in slow motion.

4. To return to starting position, gently move bent legs back to floor, one at a time.

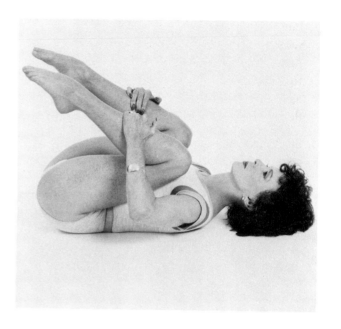

NOTE: Exercises #9 and #10 are progressive exercises designed to achieve a greater stretch. You raise your buttocks 1 inch off the floor in #9; you raise it 2 to 3 inches off in #10.

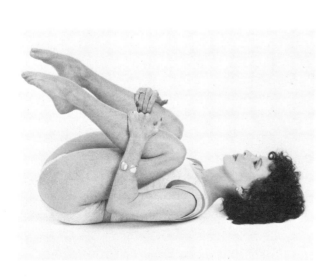

BACK STRETCH #10

1. Lie on floor, knees bent, feet on floor a hip-width apart, 1 to 1½ feet from buttocks. Arms are straight and resting on floor next to body. Stretch muscles at back of neck, as though you were going to flatten it on floor; then relax it.

2. Bring both knees up to chest and spread to shoulder-width. Grasp inside of legs below knees.

3. Gently curl up pelvis in direction of navel. Raise buttocks 2 to 3 inches off floor. Hold for a count of 5. Release slowly back to floor, one vertebra at a time. Repeat 5 times in slow motion.

4. Gently return bent legs, one at a time, to floor.

BACK STRETCH #11

1. Lie on floor, knees bent, feet on floor a hip-width apart, 1 to 1½ feet from buttocks. Arms are straight and resting on floor next to body. Stretch muscles at back of neck, as though you were going to flatten it on floor; then relax it.

2. Stretch right arm straight back over head and rest on floor. Tighten buttocks, curl up pelvis (pelvic wave). Slide right leg out straight on floor in front. Stretch arm and leg at the same time. Keep body relaxed. Hold for count of 5 to 10.

3. Return to starting position. Repeat on other side.

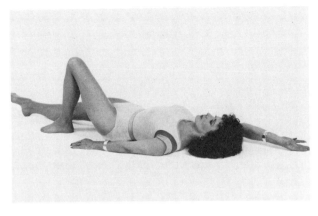

NOTE: If you wish, after this exercise, stretch opposite arms and legs at the same time, but be careful not to arch lower back.

BACK STRETCH #12

Of all the spine stretches, this is one of the greatest body-savers. I have found it to be the most effective for straightening my hips and spine. After wearing high heels (even half-inch ones), this exercise is an absolute necessity for untwisting my body and preventing me from going into spasm. It is one of the most popular of my stretches, and people all over the world have told me how it has helped their backs.

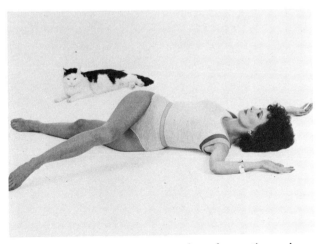

NOTE: This exercise stretches the entire spine (especially lower back), chest muscles (pectorals), side abdominals, hip and buttocks muscles, outer thighs.

1. Lie on floor, knees bent, feet on floor a hip-width apart, 1 to 1½ feet from buttocks. Arms are out at shoulder level, elbows bent at right angles, backs of hands resting on floor. Stretch muscles at back of neck, as though you were going to flatten it on floor; then relax it.

2. Lift right knee up toward chest, straighten left leg on floor (or if too difficult, keep it bent while on floor), and bring bent right leg over left leg, relaxing right foot. Allow gravity to bring knee as close to floor as possible. If your toes can touch the floor, let them. If not, just keep the right leg elevated and relaxed; the goal is eventually to have the entire bent leg rest on floor. Make sure your right shoulder and elbow remain on the floor; it is more important for the stretch in the lower back to have the shoulders on the floor than to bring the knee to the floor. Hold for count of 10 to 60.

3. In triple slow motion, keeping knee bent, bring bent right knee back to center; rest right foot on floor. Slide left leg up so that both knees are bent. Straighten right leg on floor and repeat on other side.

FINAL RELAXER

Getting up, the right way

1. Lie on floor, knees bent, feet on floor a hip-width apart, 1 to 1½ feet from buttocks. Arms are relaxed and resting on floor next to body. Stretch muscles at back of neck, as though you were going to flatten it on floor.

2. Allow bent legs to drop over to left one at a time. Slowly roll body over to rest on left side; rest head on bent arms; keep legs bent resting on each other (fetal position). Raise knees if necessary so that lower back is totally released. In this fetal position, clear your mind and let go of everything. Take this opportunity to go to your fantasy place of greatest relaxation. Now, feel yourself melting into the floor even more.

   NOTE: Use this relaxer whenever you wish.

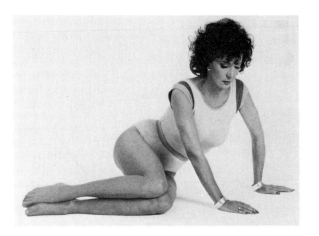

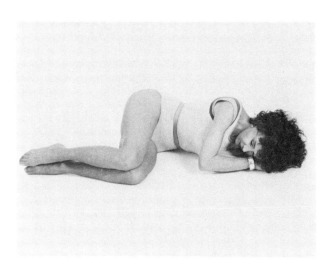

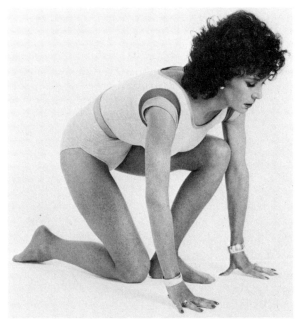

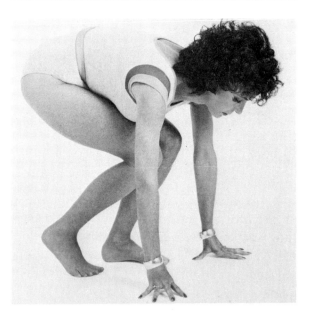

5.
Everyday Activities

As you go through the day, there are numerous ways to conserve energy and lessen the wear and tear on your body. Here are some tips to turn everyday routines into opportunities for increasing your awareness and protecting your back.

There is a wide range of exercises in this chapter. Experience as many as you can—they're all wonderful. Choose the ones that suit your needs, or do them all, or keep switching for variety.

Nothing affects the back more than the way you stand and walk and sit. It's almost a chicken-and-egg dilemma—sometimes it's difficult to say which comes first, because posture affects back health, and back health affects posture. Your posture is also a powerful nonverbal communicator. It tells the world how you feel. If you walk around slumped over, you are probably giving the appearance of carrying the weight of the world on your shoulders—something you want to avoid when walking into the room for that all-important job interview.

Unfortunately, most of us don't know how to stand or walk. True, we taught ourselves when we were babies, but through the years a combination of physical and emotional factors have influenced our posture so that it is usually necessary to relearn. Becoming aware and retraining yourself to stand, walk, and sit properly until you make it a habit is essential for everyone, but even more so for people with back problems.

STANDING

<u>Do</u>:

- Get a firm footing. Your feet are your foundation, and if your stance is not firm, the rest of your body will be unbalanced. That's why the kind of shoes you wear are so important (see page 49). Keep

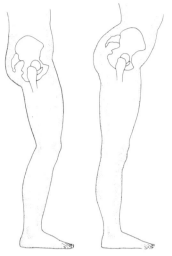

Right Way   Wrong Way

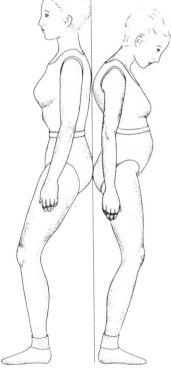

Right Way   Wrong Way

your feet comfortably apart (usually a hip-width), with knees and legs relaxed, weight evenly distributed between both sides of body and on feet. Toes should be facing front.

- Tighten buttocks and curl up pelvis (pelvic wave) slightly to keep spine stretched and as straight as possible (not bent forward or back). Think of your pelvis as a bowl filled with liquid; if you tilt it downward, the contents will spill. Shoulders should be held back and relaxed.
- Relax chest and make a conscious effort to keep shoulders down.
- Think "tall." Stretch neck up in back, pull in chin, and imagine a string attached to the top of your head pulling it (gently) toward the ceiling. Keep eyes facing front, not down.
- Whenever you have the opportunity, stand against a wall and try to push your shoulder blades flat (don't forget to do the pelvic wave).
- If you stand for a length of time, rest one foot on a low stool or chair to prevent fatigue and stiffness. Change positions often.

When I was a child I loved cowboy movies with stars like Tom Mix, Gene Autry, and Roy Rogers. They would throw open the swinging doors to the saloon as if not even lightning could touch them. They were always standing with one foot on the brass footrest, leaning their bodies over the bar. I used to think cowboys were dumb; in reality, they were quite smart. With those high-heeled boots, they were doing the best thing to relieve their lower backs. It's a shame they didn't know about the pelvic wave; but maybe they did. . . .

- Be patient. It took a long time to develop poor postural habits, and you can't expect to undo them without practice and time.
- Relax, relax, relax. You're not one of the troops being reviewed by the Commander-in-Chief. See pages 79–81 for excellent exercises you can do while standing.

<u>Don't</u>:

- Lock knees.
- Lean or slump to one side.
- Push chin and head forward, or let them slump down.
- Stand on toes or heels.
- Turn feet out or in.
- Thrust chest out.
- Hunch shoulders.
- Arch lower back.
- Allow abdominal muscles to sag or be pushed out.

WALKING

<u>Do</u>:

- Relax knees.
- Swing your leg from the hip, let your arms move naturally.
- Current medical opinion recommends taking short strides, which are more efficient than long ones and present less stress to the neck and back. Relax neck and shoulders.

- Think of your body as floating like a feather. (Thinking "up" will help counteract the tendency to come down too hard with your feet.) Enjoy yourself; walking should be a pleasurable activity.
- When climbing stairs, touch the stair with the ball of your foot and drop the heel as much as possible, then go up to the next step with the ball of the other foot. Climb with your leg muscles, not those of your back.

<u>Don't:</u>
- Walk with your knees locked.
- Lean back or too far forward.
- Walk on heels or toes only.
- Arch lower back.
- Lead with head or chin, or let head fall backward.
- Turn feet out or in.

SITTING

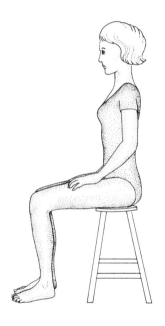

<u>Do:</u>
- Keep your knees higher than your hips. A stool or some other object is essential (try some fat telephone books). Keep your feet flat on the stool.
- Sit straight. A hard-backed chair is the best piece of furniture for this. Tightening the abdominal muscles helps to eliminate the hollow. You can also place a small cushion or folded towel behind your lower back. (I know people who have sometimes resorted to folding up a sweater or even a jacket!) Some office chairs have flexible back supports that move when you do. Sit close enough to the desk so you can lean against the chair back to support your lower back.
- Use a chair with arms so you can rest your elbows or forearms (except, of course, for typing). This helps stretch your spine and takes some of the pressure off your lower back.
- Keep feet about 1½ to 2 feet apart; this seems to be a more comfortable position than close together.
- Get up and move around as often as possible. Stiffness will set in if you stay in a sitting position too long. Try some easy stretches (see Everyday Exercises, pages 73–82).
- Practice holding your head correctly: Stretch the back of your neck as though there were strings pulling it toward the ceiling. Keep your chin pulled in and eyes facing front. If you're involved in an activity that requires reading, try to keep the reading matter at eye level.
- Learn how to get in and out of chairs. This simple movement can be a real challenge for back sufferers. To get out, place one foot in front of the other, slide your buttocks close to the edge, and with your back still straight lift yourself up using your thighs and pushing up with your arms, either against the seat or arms of the chair or on your thighs. Be sure to remain erect.
- Be aware if you're sitting more toward one side than the other. We all tend to favor one; alternate sides.

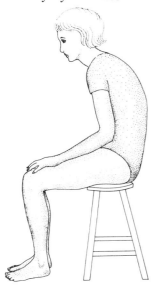

Don't:

- Slump, round your shoulders, or jut your chin out.
- Cross your legs, particularly at the knees. This causes you to become lopsided and will affect the evenness of your spine.
- Hunch your shoulders. Be aware of any tension there and keep them down. Imagine there's a weight on them.
- Lean over a desk or table; instead, keep your back straight. Depending on the type of work you do, this may not always be possible. But once you're aware, you might want to practice *in between* work periods, when you take either a breather or a full break. You will be surprised at how many opportunities you will have.

SPECIAL SITTING POSITIONS

It's good (for your back and your psyche) to make radical changes in how you sit every once in a while. Here are some suggestions:

Rockers really can relax your back, and they're very calming.

Cross-legged. Eastern people have been sitting on the floor (and even chairs) with their legs crossed in front of them for centuries.

Special chairs. There are many kinds. One popular one is tilted (without a back) so that you rest your weight on your knees (the chair is heavily padded, of course). Some people with swayback or knee problems find this chair uncomfortable.

Table heights. The next time you're in a restaurant, look around and notice how everyone is bending over to eat. This is because the height of tables has not changed for hundreds of years even though people today generally are taller. To counteract this poor posture, one has to be very conscious to sit erect, bring food up to your mouth instead of leaning over (soup is a little difficult unless you're wearing a bib). For table work, use a slanted surface, such as an artist's drawing board.

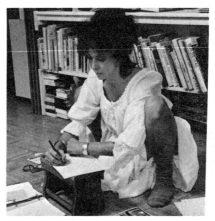
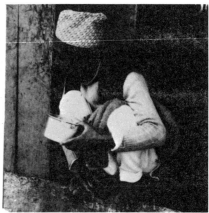

My Favorite: So called because, while writing this book, I would sit on the floor with my legs spread or sit on my haunches with my buttocks touching the floor, which I learned while living in Nepal. I don't know if you would be able to get into this position or if you would enjoy it, but it makes my back feel wonderful. I have the advantage of working at home; it may not be appropriate for an office.

Warning: Do not sit too near heels as it may be harmful to knee joints.

Watching television. Position the TV set so that you are sitting up straight, not slumping or misaligned. If you watch in bed, use a proper support for your back and neck; a bed rest, wedged pillow, neck pillow, or several regular pillows will help. Bend your knees and place a small pillow under them. You can lie on the floor and watch television as long as you have the set at eye level. This is a perfect time to do floor stretches; in fact, the entire family can get into this relaxing activity—especially the children.

Using the telephone. This ordinary activity is a killer for the neck, shoulders, and back. When *Callanetics* was published, I spent days on the phone answering questions from readers. I needed a neck brace and two arm slings—one for writing and the other for holding the phone. I really understood what secretaries and receptionists go through. For this reason, I have included a large selection of neck and shoulder exercises while sitting (see pages 75, 76, 78, 81).

Learn to hold the phone in your hand. *Never* cradle it between your shoulder and neck; this is a sure way to get a stiff neck and, with time, serious problems. If you can't use your hand to hold the phone, get a shoulder rest for it. When writing, hold the phone in one hand and write with the other. Support your arms by placing your elbows on the desk, keeping your back erect. Also, be sure to change sides frequently.

SLEEPING

POSITIONS

Side. There appears to be a consensus that the preferable sleeping position for back sufferers and for everyone who wants to protect the back is the side position. You will no doubt favor the side you are most comfortable on, but it's a good idea to alternate. If you have spasms on one side, it's a good idea to lie on the opposite side. Your knees should be bent and drawn up in a womblike position. If you wish, you may place a pillow between your knees to improve alignment and circulation; choose one that is appropriate to your size and frame. The object of lying on your side is to keep the entire spine parallel to the mattress. Both arms should be in front of your body to align your spine; and you should use a soft pillow to support your neck.

Stomach. If you're swaybacked, you should avoid sleeping on your stomach, because it increases the arch of your back and may cause you discomfort. But if you are lacking a natural lumbar curve (and if you don't have any neck problems), sleeping on the stomach is actually advisable. If you absolutely will not be comfortable in any other position, place a small pillow under your abdomen; this helps flatten low back curve. In an unconscious effort to accomplish this flattening, some people put their hands under the abdomen, which may put too much pressure on arms and hands. Finally, a pillow under your head and chest will give you more comfort, and you should try to switch sides.

Back. Sleeping on your back gives you the least mobility. Therefore, you may have a tendency to be stiff in the morning. For a variety of medical reasons (hiatal hernia, for example), some people must sleep on their back. If you have to be elevated, use a wedge under the mattress or a wedge pillow (see pages 186–187) to support the upper back and head. If you don't require elevation, you can use a small pillow under your neck. And you should have a small pillow under the thighs to keep the pelvis tilted. If your legs have to be elevated, stack several pillows under your legs and keep your knees bent; this relaxes the psoas and is excellent for swaybacked people as well as sciatica sufferers.

SURFACES

Some doctors say you must have a board under the mattress. This is so individual, and people get so dogmatic about it, that you may hear as many opinions on the type of mattress as there are mattresses. The significant issue is that the surface should be firm and not sagging. (See pages 185–186 for more information.) Some people claim they can sleep on nothing softer than a floor. What you choose will vary depending on your size, weight, and condition. You must be comfortable.

THE EVERYDAY WAKING-UP EXERCISE

While still in bed, lying on your back, bend your elbows, keeping the backs of your hands flat against the mattress. Straighten one leg; slowly bend the knee of the other leg, bring it toward your chest and then over the other leg, trying to get it to touch the mattress. Hold for as long as you wish. Then slowly bring the knee back to your chest, straighten the leg, and repeat on the other side (see page 57).

GETTING UP AND OUT OF BED

Lie on your side (with knees bent) toward the edge of the bed. Move your body as close as possible to the edge. Raise your body up to a sitting position by placing the weight of your torso on one or both hands and pushing up. Then gently bring your legs over the edge of bed, touch the floor, and stand up. If you need additional help, lift your body by placing your hands on the edge of the mattress and pushing up. To lie down, reverse the order.

MAKING A BED

If possible, while still in bed, lie on your back and pull the sheet and covers up toward you to straighten them. Then fold over corner enough to get out. When you're out, pull the corner back and don't worry about tucking in edges. To make a bed while you're not in it, avoid bending over; instead, kneel on one or both knees.

BATHROOM

We spend a great deal of time in the bathroom each day, and don't realize what harm we can do to the back in ordinary activities there. Here's your opportunity to take advantage of that time to help your back.

Toilet. The usual Western position of sitting on the toilet is the worst possible one for bad back sufferers, not to mention your bowels.

The best position can be achieved by placing your feet on a small stool so that your knees are elevated. In this position, your feet are the support for your lower back, which is curved, and your abdominal muscles are supported as well.

Basin. When you're at the basin shaving (men), brushing your teeth, washing your face, or doing any of the hundreds of things you do there, be sure to keep your knees relaxed (bent as much as possible). You should do the pelvic wave to release any tension in the lower back. What helps you achieve this is to rest one foot on a small stool, box, or—if you're flexible enough and the basin is secure!—the edge of the basin itself. If you don't use any of these aids, you should be conscientious about doing the pelvic wave and bending from the hips, not the back.

Bathing. Nothing is more relaxing than a warm soak, but don't make the water too hot, because it tires the muscles too much. Even in the tub, it is necessary to support your lower back and neck. There are special bath pillows (see pages 186–187), or you can use a folded towel under the small of your back and your upper shoulders and neck. If your tub is short, you can bend your knees or rest your feet on the rim, which will naturally tilt your pelvis and round your lower back. This is an excellent place to do some simple exercises (see pages 75–76). While you're taking a shower, you can do some neck and shoulder stretches and still soap up. Hot water showers are excellent for helping to relieve spasms or soreness. Be sure to stand on a nonslip mat.

For women, resist the temptation to shave your legs if it means you have to bend down. You can do it better with your leg raised, resting on something such as the rim of the tub, a stool, or the toilet. Better yet, sit on the closed toilet seat and rest your leg on the sink counter.

DRESSING

Who would think such a simple, unconscious activity as dressing could possibly be a problem? But it is for people with back troubles—and sometimes can even cause them. I know someone who bent down to tie his shoe and ended up flat on his back for six weeks with excruciatingly painful sciatica. Even though your mother taught you, it's important that you relearn how to dress to avoid any further back complications. Here are some tips to help you form new habits.

Tops. When putting on sweaters, dresses, etc., over your head, put arms in one at a time and be careful not to strain your neck. Try to wear garments that open all the way; short sleeves are easier than long ones.

Bras. Use front-fastening bras or turn the bra around and fasten in front.

Shoes, Pants. Always put on shoes and pants sitting down. For pants, put legs in one at a time, then stand up to finish dressing. Put on shoes one foot at a time from a sitting position, then bring foot up or stand and place your foot on chair or other elevated surface to lace.

When wearing boots, use socks with a silky texture; that way they won't cling to the boots, making them difficult to take off. Avoid boots that are too tight.

Pantyhose, exercise tights, body stockings, girdles

Put all of these on and take them off with extreme care. Do not wear them if they are too tight; even putting them on sitting down can impose too much pressure on your lower back. I knew a girl who went into spasm just from wriggling herself into a pair of exercise tights.

LIFTING AND CARRYING

There is probably no greater assault to the back than improper lifting and carrying of heavy objects. The following suggestions apply not only to loads that are heavy; you should use extreme care in lifting and carrying anything—from a valise to a baby.

LIFTING FROM BELOW

<u>Do:</u>

- Test the weight of an object before lifting it; weight is often deceiving. If you squat down (with legs apart and one behind the other), and judge the weight by lifting it slowly with your hands, you will have a better idea of how to do it while avoiding any possible injury to your back.
- Keep a straight back; never round it or bend over.

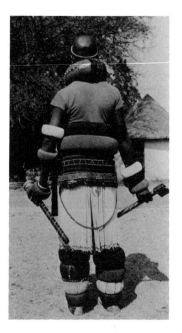

Body weights: This woman was married. The circular weights hanging on her body were her marriage rings. This particular tribe wound rope-covered metal on a bride; smaller rings went up the leg, covering the knees. I was told that this was to prevent the bride from running away from her husband if he beat or abused her. It was impossible to run with all that weight, and the knees didn't bend. So when the women picked up something from the ground, they had to spread their legs like a giraffe drinking at a water hole, bending from the hips and bringing the torso forward and down. To come back up, they had to lock their knees and bring the torso straight up to a standing position, putting incredible pressure on their lower back (especially with the extra weight on their body). Notice how her right shoulder is higher than her left. Soon the rings are going to be resting at an angle. I don't have a clue why she always carried a carved stick and a stone hatchet.

- Bend your knees; if necessary, squat down on one knee. You want to lower your center of gravity so that the lifting can be done with your legs—taking advantage of some of the strongest muscles of the body—not your back.
- Get close to the object; this will prevent you from bending over.
- Tighten your buttocks and curl up your pelvis (pelvic wave—see pages 88–90) for the duration of the lift. If the object is particularly heavy, and you have a midway place to rest it, you may want to do the lift in stages. To do this, put the object down at a higher level, take a breather, do the pelvic wave again, and then continue. Use your legs to assist the lift.
- Raise your body as a unit; do not bend at the waist.
- Keep your feet flat on the floor.
- Move slowly and carefully.
- Get assistance if the load is too heavy; this is no time for macho or foolhardy behavior.

<u>Don't</u>:
- Lift anything in front of you higher than your waistline.
- Bend over to lift heavy objects.
- Make sudden, fast, or jerking movements.
- Attempt to lift or carry anything heavy if your back is in pain.

LIFTING FROM ABOVE

<u>Do</u>:
- Try to avoid this by keeping heavy objects on shelves between waist and shoulder height.
- Always use a step stool if you must lift something stored above shoulder level; this will help prevent your back from arching.
- Keep buttocks tightened and pelvis curled up if you must lift a heavy object to a level at or above shoulder height.
- Use your arms to lift, not your back.

<u>Don't</u>:
- Stand on your tiptoes.
- Arch your back; reaching overhead causes you to hyperextend. Be conscious of movements that are causing your back to arch and correct them immediately.

LIFTING FROM A CAR

When lifting something heavy from a car trunk or truck, move the object to the edge, lean against the car, bend knees, tilt pelvis up, and use your legs for the lift. Avoid any twisting motions.

CARRYING

It is necessary here to repeat the precaution against carrying anything heavy unless your back is free of pain. If you are experi-

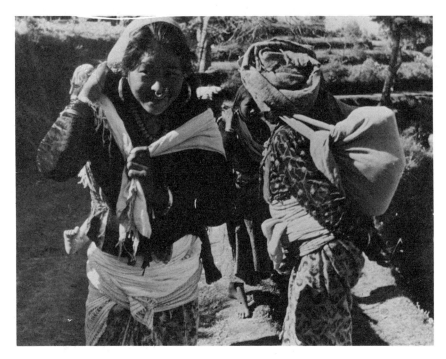

Travel: While trekking to Mount Everest from Katmandu (which took about nine days), I was followed by these young women. The babies strapped on their backs never cried. When they breast-fed their babies, the mothers kept walking—they had a unique way of twisting their bodies and flipping the babies forward in front of them without missing one step. They were barefoot, climbing mountain after mountain, no warm cloth to cover them in the freezing nights.

encing problems with your back, any weight-bearing activity will aggravate the problems. Don't do it; let someone else do it.

<u>Do:</u>
- Keep the object as close as possible to your body, either at chest or waist level in front. Tighten your buttocks and curl up your pelvis (pelvic wave), and try not to round your shoulders. This helps to distribute the weight and take pressure off the back. When carrying luggage or shopping bags, you can improve the situation if you distribute the weight evenly on both sides.
- Carry heavy objects on your shoulders. It's better for your back when the muscles push up toward a weight than pull down.
- Try to keep your body straight. There's a tendency when you're carrying something heavy on one side to lean over to that side. This creates an imbalance in the body, and possibly related pain. For this reason, it's better to wear a backpack, which distributes the weight across both shoulders, than a shoulder bag carried on only one shoulder.
- Bend your knees; this helps take some of the weight off the back and makes walking with a heavy load much easier.

<u>Don't:</u>
- Bend over the object you are carrying or allow your back to round; keep it straight.
- Lean or tilt over to one side; if the object is on one side, counteract

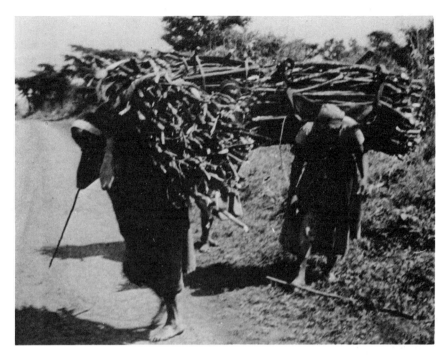

Carrying: It takes these elderly Kenyan women from sunrise to sunset to walk miles from their village and back. They collect the wood, cut it a certain length, remove branches, leaves, and twigs, pile it up, rope it—and complete the incredible task of hoisting the heavy pile on their backs, where it is balanced and secure enough to keep in place for the long journey at sunset.

the force by leaning slightly to the other side to keep your body even.
• Lock your knees.
• Let your abdominal muscles slacken.

A word about handbags: Although shoulder bags are very popular and convenient, they present problems. Usually, they place too much weight on the shoulder, so they are best worn slung over the shoulder and across the body, resting on the opposite hip. By all means switch sides as much as possible.

BENDING

Most of us are unaware of how much we bend throughout the day. As in lifting and carrying, there is an art to bending. Always bend your knees (do not bend over with straight legs) and get down as close to what you're doing as possible. If you're doing something such as scrubbing the floor, get down on all fours. Keep your back straight; don't bend over or slump.

PULLING AND PUSHING

Both these activities are strenuous when you are dealing with heavy loads. When possible, it's better to push than pull because pulling puts more stress on the back. Again, bend deeply and get a firm footing; keep feet apart and weight evenly distributed over them. Face the object. Keep your back straight, tighten your buttocks, and curl up your pelvis. Use your arms and legs, not your back, to do the pushing or pulling. Do not strain; move slowly and don't jerk.

TRAVELING

People don't realize what a strain travel can be and how much stress it places on the back in particular. From getting to your means of transportation to sleeping in unfamiliar beds with the wrong (usually foam rubber) pillows, it's a nightmare from beginning to end.

I find plane travel the worst. First there's the trauma of getting to the airport, always through the worst traffic (don't forget your neck exercises—see page 75). Then there's the inevitable fact of life from which no one is spared, these days: waiting in the airport. One can learn more about what not to do sitting in the terminal and watching people getting on and off planes. I've seen so many people with such an incredible amount of baggage (with goodness knows what's in it) hanging off their bodies that I can actually feel the strain in *my* neck and lower back. You would think the government had said, "Evacuate the country, take what you need for the rest of your life and only what you can carry on your person."

I'm always amazed at the women in high heels, with all manner of bags hanging off them, running to catch planes. But I'm totally awe-struck when I see a pregnant woman in high heels, carrying a baby, trailing two other children (with a leash attached to one child's wrist to prevent him from running away), pushing a cart filled with heavy luggage and running. That's enough to put anyone into spasm!

If you have one carry-on article (even a handbag), don't hang it on your shoulder. Instead, carry it in front of your chest, supported by both bent arms. Keep switching sides of anything you are carrying.

Weight of luggage can be very deceiving. When you first pick up something, it may not feel so heavy. But try this simple test before you start lugging it around: Lift it to shoulder level with your elbow bent and hold it there for sixty seconds. This is guaranteed to make you conscious of what it will do to your lower back; if it becomes too heavy just using your arm, imagine what it will do to your neck and back! Perhaps you could manage if you walked only about three feet carrying heavy luggage, but in some airports it seems as though you have to walk as much as three miles on something called carpet, which feels like concrete, or concrete itself.

This is where luggage carriers come in. I have found they are essential. (Unfortunately, I'm one of those people who carries an excessive amount of hand luggage—with leotards, makeup, etc.—in case my checked baggage gets lost and I am left stranded before a TV appearance. The newer carts have small wheels instead of large ones, which makes them less clumsy. If you use rectangular-shaped bags and place them on the cart lengthwise, you will be able to get through even the narrowest aisles with these carts. Then you can roll your stuff all over the airport, through the gate, and onto the plane without having to lift them (this isn't too difficult if you squat down to undo the elastic cord, but it's even better not to use a cord at all) except to go through the X-ray machine checking for grenades, zap guns, etc. What's more, while you're standing in line, you can put one foot on the carrier to relieve your back. And remember: It is better for your back to push rather than pull.

When you get to your seat, don't attempt to lift the bags into the overhead rack. Instead, say to someone, "Excuse me. I have a very bad back. Could you possibly put this up for me, please?" You would be surprised how terribly kind and considerate most people are about assisting.

Upon landing, you may have to wait until everyone disembarks to repack your cart. Although it seems like a nuisance, it is worth the effort to save your back.

Now, about the seats. Airplane seats were not designed for human rears. If you have a bad back, try to at least get a window seat, so if you fall asleep your head will rest against something solid and not hang over the aisle. Of course, you must put a pillow between your head and the window. In fact, immediately after getting your bags in place, find two pillows before they are all gone. Roll up one (or a blanket) and place it on the lower back where it feels best. If it's impossible to get either a pillow or blanket, you can use a rolled-up sweater. The idea is to sit up as straight as possible with your lower back pressed flat against the back of the seat. With the other pillow for your head (there are inflatable neck pillows that are excellent for traveling; see pages 186–187) you should be prepared for a comfortable takeoff and flight. As for the landing, do the same—but good luck! Landings are really hard on the vertebrae. Sometimes it helps to drop your head between your knees while landing.

Driving a car presents a major challenge for the back. Again, the key is to sit as straight as possible. There are several kinds of backrests that you can buy (see pages 186–187). In place of one, you can use a cushion or a rolled-up towel. If your car has a headrest, learn how to adjust it to give your neck support. Adjust your seat to the most forward comfortable position; your knees should be well bent and higher than your hips. Driving can be hazardous; in a study some years ago, people who spent a great deal of time driving were found to be very susceptible to ruptured discs—truck drivers, to an even greater extent (about five times more often). Remember to do your neck exercises when you're stuck in traffic and make sure to stop every hour or so to walk around or stretch.

6.

Everyday Exercises

When I was living in and traveling around India, I could only afford third-class train transportation, which was a free-for-all. The other passengers who could only afford this class were the "untouchables," and I presume I was one as well. It didn't faze me one bit having to sleep on a luggage rack, barely one foot from the ceiling. I didn't feel guilty about taking up the space; there was plenty of room because no one had any luggage. Once I situated myself, lying on my back, I would have to remain in that position for eight to ten hours. It was impossible to lie on my side as there wasn't enough height for a shoulder. There was a sign that read, OCCUPANCY FOR 15 PERSONS ONLY. When I looked down at the people, they looked like little bubbles in a square container. One time I counted sixty heads (not including infants, wrapped around mothers' necks) in the compartment, plus bodies in the aisles. Naturally, there was no air-conditioning, but the windows were open to keep you from suffocating and breathing in the foul air. My face was black from the smoke of the engine. Amazingly, the people squeezed together did not seem affected by the conditions. For instance, the only way to get to the bathroom was to leap or step over the "bubbles." Consequently, no one went.

I stayed on the rack, because if I attempted to get down, I could have crushed at least five heads in the process. So I lay there in my little heaven, feeling blessed, for at least I could straighten out my legs!

From this vantage point, I watched as some people would try to move their arms, shoulders, heads, and legs, while others would try to move their hands enough to massage the feet or legs of the stranger close enough to crush them. At first it looked as though they were choreographing some bizarre dance ritual. Only later, when my own stiffness or lack of movement hit me, did I realize these strange

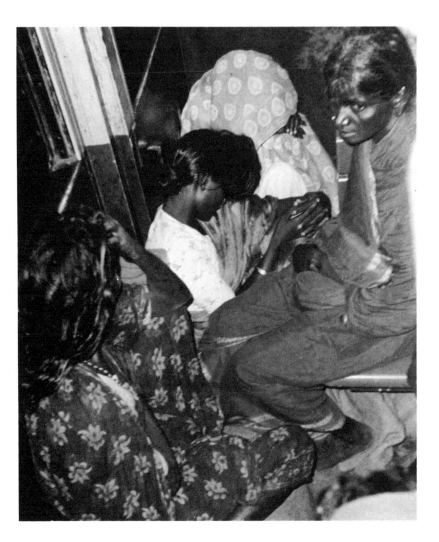

movements were a sad attempt to relieve cramped limbs and get circulation moving.

Now, when I have to wait in terminals, I often reflect on how graciously those poor people accepted their situation and tried to deal with it in the best way they could. We might not be as cramped, yet one still has to wait and often remain seated uncomfortably for hours, strapped in during long plane, bus, or car rides.

Here are some suggestions to help relieve the discomfort and anxiety that come from remaining in static positions—whether at home, at work, or while traveling—for long periods of time.

EXERCISES FOR CLOSE QUARTERS

In the workplace—whether home, office, school, or assembly line—it is essential that you move and stretch to reduce stress, gain energy, and feel relaxed.

The following exercises can be done in close quarters such as cars, buses, and planes, either sitting or standing.

NECK

NOTE: All neck exercises should be done in triple slow motion and only when you have time to relax.

Exercise 1. Slowly lower head forward and hold for 15 to 30 seconds. Slowly return to neutral position.

Exercise 2. Slowly turn head first to one side and then to the other. Hold at each side 15 to 30 seconds.

Exercise 3. Sit or stand with legs a hip-width apart, knees slightly bent. Tighten buttocks and do pelvic wave as much as possible (see pages 91–93), keeping shoulders down and chin pulled in. Slowly lower head to right so that right ear is as close as possible to right shoulder. Hold for a count of 5 to 20. Slowly return to center, stretch neck up, and repeat on other side.

Exercise 4. Begin in same position as #3. Slowly lower head to right shoulder, then gently press with left hand toward right shoulder. Hold for a count of 5 to 20. With hand, slowly return head to center, stretch neck up, and repeat on other side.

Exercise 5. Begin in same position as #3. Stretch neck up and turn head halfway between center and right shoulder, allowing gravity to pull head down. Hold for a count of 5 to 20. Gently lift head, return to center, and repeat on other side.

Exercise 6. Begin in same position as #3. Stretch neck up, then turn head extremely slowly to right, trying to look over shoulder. Hold for a count of 5 to 20. Gently return to center and repeat on other side.

Exercise 7. Begin in same position as #3. Stretch neck up and slowly lower chin toward chest. Gently move chin toward right shoulder, gradually raising it until nose is over middle of shoulder, then continue to turn head until looking over right shoulder and hold for a count of 5. Slowly lower chin to chest and repeat on left side.

Exercise 8. Begin in same position as #3. Stretch neck up and place either hand (fingers pointing downward) on base of skull. Gently press head down toward chest with hand. Hold for a count of 5. Keeping hand in place, release pressure and slowly bring head to upright position.

Exercise 9. Stand or sit with legs comfortably apart and head erect, chin pulled in. Place palm of right hand gently against right side of head. Try to turn head to right as you gently press (resist) head toward center. Hold for a count of 3 to 5. Repeat on other side.

Exercise 10. Stand or sit with legs comfortably apart and head erect, chin pulled in. Place both palms on front of forehead and push head gently against them. Hold for a count of 3 to 5. Now place hands on neck at base of head, with elbows out to side. Push head gently against hands. Hold for count of 3 to 5.

SHOULDERS/ARMS

Exercise 1. Place right hand on left shoulder, keeping right elbow up. With left hand push elbow gently toward left shoulder (right hand will slide toward back of left shoulder). Repeat on other side.

Exercise 2. Place right hand behind right shoulder and with left hand gently push right upper arm up and toward back. Repeat on other side.

Exercise 3. Bring right arm up, bend elbow, and rest hand on shoulder blade. Bring left hand behind back and up to try to make hands meet. Do not force stretch. Hold for a count of 5. Release gently and repeat on other side.

Exercise 4. Raise right shoulder up to right ear, then lower. Do 5 times, then repeat on other side.

Exercise 5. Raise right shoulder up to right ear; rotate in a circular motion 5 times; reverse direction and repeat with left shoulder.

Exercise 6. Bend forward from hips and gently try to get elbows and shoulder blades to touch behind you. (If you feel you are arching lower back, do a small pelvic wave.)

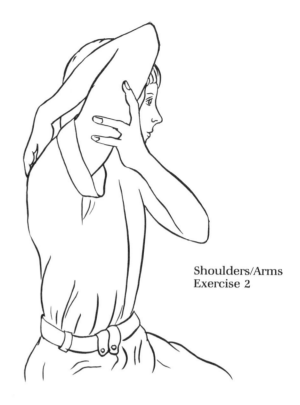

Shoulders/Arms
Exercise 2

Shoulders/Arms
Exercise 3

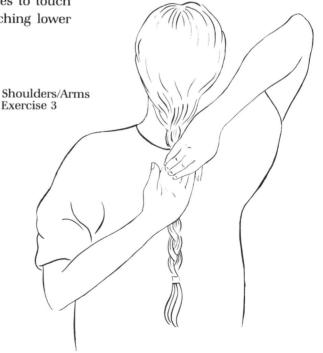

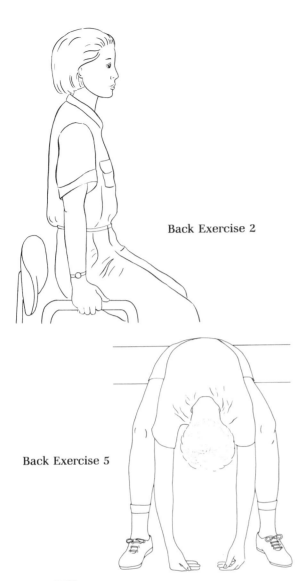

Back Exercise 2

Back Exercise 5

BACK

Exercise 1. Do pelvic wave (see pages 88–90).

Exercise 2. In a chair with armrests, keeping spine straight and chin pulled in, lift up body by pressing hands against arms of chairs. Hold for as long as you want (this helps relieve buttocks fatigue).

When your wrists are strong enough, once you have lifted yourself, you can do the pelvic wave or pelvic rotations (see pages 88–95, 132–136).

Exercise 3. Keeping hips forward, hands resting on thighs, twist upper body from waist slowly to right and then to left.

Exercise 4. Touch left elbow to right knee, bringing right knee up and stretching your back. Repeat on other side.

Exercise 5. Lean forward from hips and let head drop gently between knees, arms to floor. Relax neck and stretch lower back. Return to sitting one vertebra at a time (do not tighten lower back).

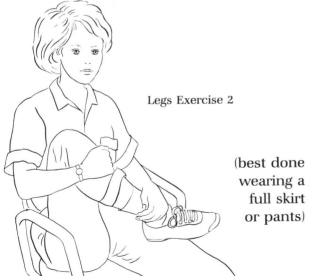

Legs Exercise 2

(best done wearing a full skirt or pants)

LEGS

Exercise 1. Sit erect in chair with knees bent. Bring right leg up, hug toward chest with both hands, and hold for a count of 5 to 20. If you wish, rotate ankles 5 times in each direction before repeating on other side.

Exercise 2. With right hand, bring right leg up toward chest, place left hand on ankle, and pull leg gently toward body. Hold for a count of 5 to 20. Gently release leg and repeat on other side.

> *If you're stuck in a car in traffic, remember to do neck exercises, pelvic wave, and anything else you have room for. Be conscious not to clench jaw, hunch shoulders, tighten lower back.*

ADDITIONAL SITTING ROUTINES

SHOULDERS

Exercise 1. Sitting straight, bring both arms over head, turn palms to face ceiling, and lace fingers together. Stretch arms as high as possible. Release and repeat several times.

Exercise 2. Sitting as straight as possible, place both hands behind head, elbows to side. Keeping chin pulled in and back of neck straight, slowly try to get elbows to touch each other behind you. Hold for a count of 15; then bring back to center and, rounding head forward slightly, gently try to get elbows to touch in front of you. Hold for a count of 15.

Exercise 3. Sitting as straight as possible, clasp hands behind back, then slowly and gently try to raise arms as high as possible behind you. Keep chin pulled in and back of neck stretched.

BACK

Exercise 1. Bend from hips and lower head slowly between knees, grasp inside ankles, bend elbows all the way to the side, and round back like a cat, feeling the stretch. To come up to sitting erect, straighten up one vertebra at a time.

Exercise 2. Place feet a shoulder-width apart, bend from the hips, and touch left foot with right hand, bringing left arm up straight behind you. Without sitting up, repeat on other side.

Exercise 3. Sit in a swivel chair with forearms and elbows resting on desk in front of you (or on arms of chair). Keeping your upper body straight and feet flat on floor about a hip-width apart, swivel to right, center, and left. When returning to center, tighten buttocks and do pelvic wave, releasing as you go to either side. Be careful not to push abdomen out, arch back, or move knees.

Exercise 4. Sit in a chair with hands gently resting on back of neck, elbows out to side, feet a hip-width apart. Pressing spine against back of chair, do pelvic wave and curl upper body. Keeping chin tucked in and back of neck stretched, gently aim nose toward chest. Do not strain or arch neck.

The important point to remember is that keeping the body in motion lubricates the joints, keeping you more limber and feeling younger. Do not *arch lower back*

STANDING

What follows are specific standing exercises. Throughout the day, you have many opportunities to do them, particularly while waiting on lines for buses, movies, tables, etc.

When you have more room, use your imagination to take advantage of doorways and secure countertops (sinks, desks, tables) to do the following stretches. Outdoors, you can use fences, trees, playground equipment, stop signs, parking meters, even telephone poles if you're careful about splinters.

BACK

Exercise 1. Stand erect with feet a hip-width apart, knees slightly bent. Move right hip out to the side as far as possible and then up toward the ceiling. Hold for a count of 15. Repeat on left side.

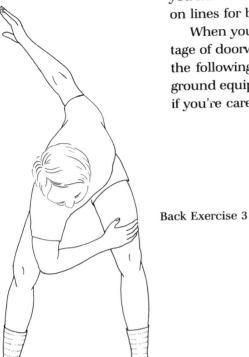

Back Exercise 3

Exercise 2. Stand erect with legs a hip-width apart and arms stretched toward ceiling or resting on top of hip bones. Bend knees and slowly move right hip out to right side as far as possible. Do pelvic wave (see pages 88–93) as you rotate hips toward front, then to left side, and back to starting position; don't stick out buttocks. Repeat in each direction a few times. This relaxes and limbers lower back and hip joints.

Exercise 3. Stand with bent knees a hip- or shoulder-width apart, whichever feels more comfortable. Tighten buttocks and curl up pelvis (pelvic wave). Lean upper torso forward and place right hand on left leg above knee. Push right elbow against inside of right knee and move left arm straight out behind you as far as possible. Hold for a count of 15 to 30. Stay in same crouched position and repeat on left side. Release arms and return to standing position, one vertebra at a time, straightening legs last.

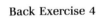

Back Exercise 4

Exercise 4. Stand with back to fence or wall, about 1 to 2 feet away, feet a shoulder-width apart, knees bent, and toes facing forward. Slowly turn upper torso toward wall and place hands on wall at shoulder height. Hold for a count of 15. Return to center and repeat on other side. Twist only upper body; *try to keep hips straight and facing front.*

(continued)

BACK, *continued*

Exercise 5. Stand with arms behind you, almost shoulder level, holding on to a door frame. Tighten buttocks and do pelvic wave, bend knees slightly, and lean body forward away from door. Try to keep upper back straight. See illustration, page 27.

Exercise 6. With arms straight, hold on to edge of desk, sink, counter, or any stable furniture. Pull torso away from edge, aiming buttocks toward floor. Bend knees and do pelvic wave. Hold for a count of 5 to 10. Then, if you wish, slowly move hips, one at a time, toward ceiling, maintaining the pelvic wave. Hold for a count of 5 to 10, then release. See page 20, Exercise 1.

Exercise 7. I always take the opportunity to do this one at the bank or while shopping. Rest bent elbows and forearms on top of counter, desk, table, etc. Slowly bend right knee. Keeping other leg straight but not locked, tighten buttocks and do pelvic wave. Feel the stretch in the lower back. Repeat on left side.

Exercise 8. Stand sideways next to wall or door at arm's length away. Straighten right arm and place palm against wall at shoulder height. Relax knees and do pelvic wave. Keep body erect. Very slowly turn entire body as a unit and walk feet to the left and around toward back until you feel stretch across chest and upper arm. Hold for a count of 10 to 20. Slowly return to original position and repeat on other side.

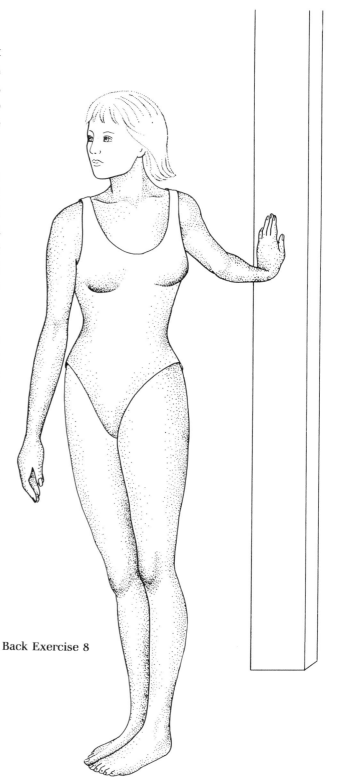

Back Exercise 8

Elevator Exercise 1

Elevator Exercise 2

ELEVATOR STRETCHES FOR THE BACK

A ride in an elevator can be a painful experience if you're having serious back pain. First of all, there's the fear that your spine may be crushed by the closing door, because you can't move quickly enough to get in and out in time. The following stretches may provide some relief; they can be done to stretch your back any time you're in an elevator or against a wall.

Exercise 1. Stand with back, head, and neck against wall or door, feet about 6 inches away. Flattening lower back as much as possible against wall, slide down wall until knees are slightly bent. Do pelvic wave. Hold for a count of 5 to 15, release pelvic wave, and slowly slide back to standing position.

Exercise 2. If you're alone in the elevator, you can do this variation: Round upper torso toward knees and rest hands on thighs above knees. Hold for a count of 15 to 30. Return to standing very slowly (by walking hands up thighs if necessary), sliding body up against the wall until you are erect. When you start to appreciate the release in the lower back, you can very delicately do the pelvic wave while still resting hands on thighs, as you press against wall.

SHOULDERS

   NOTE: The following exercise is excellent if there has been an injury or a condition such as bursitis.

Exercise 1. Stand facing wall or door, about 12 inches away. Slowly walk fingers of each hand up the wall as high as you can and then down again. (You can also do this exercise standing with side to wall.)

Exercise 2. Stand with arms straight out to sides at shoulder level. Slowly rotate arms in circular motion forward and then backward 5 to 10 times. Do not hunch shoulders.

LYING DOWN

Although you will probably have less opportunity to use these exercises, lying-down motions are good to know. Certainly, if you work at home or in a private office, you will welcome them for the relief and relaxation they afford.

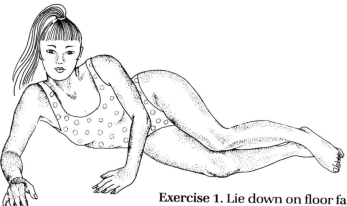

Exercise 1. Lie down on floor facing a chair, knees bent and lower legs resting on chair seat. Upper back and head may be supported by a pillow (triangular or wedge pillow is best for this—see pages 186–187); if necessary, place a small pillow or folded towel under buttocks. Pull chin in and relax in this position for as long as you can; even a few minutes can provide wonderful relief and relaxation.

Note: You can rest like this without pillows. If you do not use anything under your buttocks, lie with buttocks close to legs of chair (or under chair), resting lower legs on chair. This position is so soothing for back suffers that some people even take naps in it.

Exercise 2. Lie down, knees bent, feet on floor a hip-width apart and 1 to 1½ feet from buttocks. Rest arms on floor with elbows bent at right angles and backs of hands resting on floor. Stretch back of neck against floor. Bring legs up one at a time to chest and gently roll them, one at a time, over to right side and toward head, trying to keep shoulders on floor. Hold for a count of 5. Bring legs back to center, one at a time, and repeat on other side.

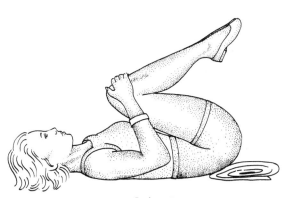

Lying Down Exercise 3

Exercise 3. Lie down and place small rolled-up towel (not too thick) under tailbone. Bend knees and place feet on floor a hip-width apart. Grasp front of legs below knees and slowly bring knees to chest. Hold for as long as you want and melt into the floor. Return legs to floor, one at a time, keeping knees bent. Relax neck.

7.

Three Stages of Callanetics

Peeople with back problems, due to mental stress or physical injury, are often told not to do any exercise. Yet more than 80 percent of pain in the lower back is caused by weak or tense muscles—which means that if you *do* exercise, you should be able to relieve your back pain considerably. Furthermore, while you're in pain and terrified to move for fear of more pain, what do you do about keeping strong, maintaining a high energy level, preventing muscle atrophy or just getting through the day? How do you learn how to protect your back? You do *not* have to give up a tight, fit body because of an aching back. My first book, *Callanetics*, outlined a way to help people look ten years younger in ten hours by following a program of carefully constructed exercises. This section is designed to instruct you in basic Callanetics regardless of age or most back problems. The exercises are divided into three stages: The first is for people who are in spasm or other severe discomfort. The second and third stages are described below.

The first-stage exercises were derived from my own experience with back problems when I was so dumb that I wore heels all the time (I sometimes even slept in them!). I was already teaching Callanetics, and certainly should have known better. But the heels were a symbol to me of modern Western clothes; and it was extremely important for my emotional survival, upon returning from my eleven-year sojourn, to look like the image I had of every American female. I was in such spasm from high heels that the fear of exercising or of *any* type of body motion could actually make me feel as though I might go into deeper spasm. I would pray to God to be gentle and kind and not allow me to sneeze or cough. The only physical movement my body was capable of handling was the welling up of tears from such excruciating pain. That's how incapacitated I was! Eventually I realized that I had only two choices—to lie there and atrophy or attempt some sort of exercise. But when I attempted to do Callanetics, I could do only the most elementary motions. It is these elementary motions that I have incorporated into the first-stage exercises. I am convinced from doing them myself and teaching them to other people in pain that these first-stage movements will relieve some or all of your discomfort, as well as strengthening your body and keeping it straight and beautiful.

I have not had a back spasm for ten years, but I will never forget that excruciating pain. That spasm lasted for months, but it seemed like five years. I see no reason anyone else has to go through it.

I believe that something must be done immediately to relieve a spasm, rather than waiting for it to go away by itself. Why lie in bed in pain for days when, in most cases, you can experience immediate relief? These first-stage movements can be your initial step to that relief. Of course, you don't have to be going into or coming out of spasm to do these wonderful exercises. They are beneficial at *any time*.

The second-stage exercises are for people who can do a little more movement, and can do the first stage with ease. The third stage is for those who are still more limber; and the final exercises in this chapter are some of the actual Callanetics for strengthening and stretching specific parts of the body while protecting the back.

The stages called Callanetics are designed to teach you a technique that will make it possible for you to never again have to put pressure on your back. You will learn how to contract specific muscle areas while relaxing your back and your entire body. Most of the exercises actually stretch the spine at the same time they strengthen and stretch other muscles. Usually these are the muscles which can relieve the work load placed on the lower back. When muscles are weak or are pushed beyond their capabilities, they tire easily and are unable to do the work demanded of them. It is then that the muscles of your lower back begin to take over, resulting in stress to that area.

This can be remedied with the right kind of strengthening. For example: When the muscles surrounding and connected to the pelvis and the lower spine are equally developed, the lower back will be better protected. We all now know that we must strengthen the abdominal muscles to help relieve lower back discomfort. However, for me, that's just part of the picture. I believe all muscles from head to toe play a very important role in supporting the lower back, and for this reason my program includes exercises that strengthen all of them.

The expression "strengthen your back" has always presented a real problem for me because it seems as though I'm forever being told by doctors that my back muscles are extremely strong. I don't have to strengthen my back any more than it is already because doing my Callanetics exercises over the years has sufficiently strengthened the muscles of my back. In addition, the back gets strong from all the moving, bending, reaching, etc., of everyday life.

Your back is working long hours. It's overtaxed and overtensed. What it needs is not strengthening, but s-t-r-e-t-c-h-i-n-g. It needs to be more supple, more relaxed. I feel that the majority of other current exercise routines that supposedly "strengthen the back" actually put stress on the back.

It might help to think of these stages in the following way:

Stage I is the warm-up.

Stage II is the build-up.

Stage III is the healing.

Callanetics is the guarantee.

GUIDELINES

The following will help you do the exercises correctly without fear or injury, and will help define some of the terms used in the instructions.

• The most important first step is to become conscious of **your body** and to realize that, like it or not, it is your very own. Every body is different due to a variety of factors such as heredity, the amount and type of activity you do and have done, and how you handle stress. Learn to enjoy your uniqueness. As you do each motion, concentrate on it to **sense** the contraction and relaxation of the muscles. It is important to understand, by feeling, the difference between a relaxed muscle and one that is tensed. Muscles that are held in tension too long due to everyday stress may eventually become damaged.

Be conscious of what your muscles are communicating to you. They will tell you whether you're doing too much or too little. You're going to have to discover this for yourself; what is pain to one person is not necessarily pain to another.

Pain is often a state of mind. And the fear of it is sometimes worse than the pain itself. I find when I teach new students, some of them automatically say, "That hurts." I say to them, "What does the word *hurt* mean to you?" A few say "an injury," but about 95 percent of them say "pain." To me, feeling my muscles work is not pain at all; rather it is a beautiful sensation rushing through my body. When they understand what I'm saying (by experiencing the exercises), within minutes they change their thinking from negative to positive. Perhaps if you, too, begin to think about what you refer to as "pain" while exercising, you may suddenly discover that when you use a muscle in a new way or stretch one that hasn't been stretched in a long time (or ever) that it is not painful at all, but rather a wonderful sensation that is serving your body. When you arrive at this realization, you are truly listening to your body and are ready to take full responsibility for it. Naturally, if a motion still hurts, despite your new mind-set, stop doing it and return to an easier position.

It's normal to feel a stretching sensation when you exercise, which some of you may perceive as a slight ache, but it should not be sharp or sudden; and you should not have any trouble breathing. If you have to alter a movement in order to be comfortable, by all means do it; these directions are not carved in stone. Accept that there's only one of you in the world, and make these exercises fit your range and ability.

- Just as "No pain, no gain" is outdated (thank goodness), so is the bouncing and jerking common to the old exercises we all did in gym class (and many still do). When a direction says "Move," the movements should be **slow, smooth, and small**—no more than $\frac{1}{16}$ to $\frac{1}{4}$ inch from a neutral position.

- When a direction says "Hold for a count of 5," you should count "one one-thousand" "two one-thousand," etc., for each count.

- Breathe naturally. Don't make it an issue, but don't forget to breathe, either. If you count out loud, it helps you to breathe naturally. As a general rule, inhale before the movement and exhale slowly during the movement. I do not stress breathing in the directions; in my fifteen years of teaching, I have found that if I do, most people start to concentrate on their breathing and begin to tense their bodies, especially their backs. As a result, they usually don't learn to relax or be in control of the motions; the motions control them.

- Never lock your knees or your elbows. Holding the leg or arm straight does not mean you have to lock the knee or elbow. Just relax, relax, relax. Feel your entire body from your toes to the top of your head become wax, melting into the floor. The more you relax your entire body, the more pressure you can take off your neck and lower back. Relaxing like this gives you a wonderful opportunity to start changing your "Woe is me" negative thinking to "I'm in control of my life" positive thinking.

- Don't push your muscles at first. Always work at your own pace. Do only as many repetitions as are comfortable. *If a direction says "Move for a count of 5" or "Hold for a count of 5" and you can do only two, then do only two.* Next time you'll probably be able to do three or more. If you can do more than a direction calls for with ease, do it. Every movement builds on the previous one; eventually you will be able to contract and stretch muscles with ease. Remember that it took many years for your body to be in the limited state it is now; you can't expect to correct it overnight. One of the most common errors people make is to be too zealous. They overexert the muscle and push their bodies too hard and too soon. They mistakenly think, "If I do a few more now, I'll get stronger faster." You'll be less prone to injuries if you take the motions at your own pace and don't mimic anyone—including the instructor. Also, if you're in spasm, be extremely careful before attempting *any* body motions.

• You'll see the term *triple slow motion* in many of the following exercises. Picture a scene in a movie in slow motion. Now make the scene move even slower. This will make you aware of how slowly and gently you should move your body while doing the motions. Jerking, bouncing, jumping, and thrusting should be avoided by anyone but an athlete professionally trained in an activity that requires these specific movements.

• If you want to move to music, make sure it's soft and soothing so you feel calm and able to concentrate. Jerky music such as rock and roll has a terrible effect on most people's nervous system, and it can encourage jerky motions and losing control.

• *Warm-up* means different things to different people. The purpose of warming up is to raise the body's temperature and consequently that of the muscles. When muscles are warm, they become more pliable and will work with greater ease. Elaborate warm-ups are not necessary for these exercises; but if you're planning to do them directly after getting up in the morning, take a warm shower or move around a bit, or if you are confined to a lying-down position, try gently activating your muscles by contracting and relaxing them. For example: Starting with your toes, squeeze them as hard as possible, then slowly relax them to the same count. What you're aiming for is a warm, alive feeling in your muscles and joints.

• My exercises are not limited to either the contraction or the stretching of muscles. They form a total system, incorporating both, so they can serve as the only form of exercise you need for strengthening and shaping your body (unless you are a professional athlete).

All of these stages can be done as a separate series of exercises. I suggest that you start with the first stage so that you can discover for yourself at which level you should begin, and do only as many repetitions as are comfortable. I have also included alternatives (most of which can be done entirely on the floor) for those of you who would be most comfortable in that position. Give yourself enough time (at least ten to twenty minutes a day to start) and peace (try to turn off the telephone). Make sure you read the directions completely so you have a clear idea of how to proceed; I don't want you to have to stop in the middle of a motion to read what comes next.

Now you're ready to begin looking and feeling better, younger, and tighter than you could ever imagine. You will also have the stamina to match your looks. My hope is that you will gain enough confidence and trust in your body to let go of the fear of pain. You *can* exercise and be in total control of the well-being of your back—not at its mercy!

NOTE: Those of you familiar with my first book will notice that the sequence of Callanetics exercises here has been slightly altered. This was done to accommodate people who are in discomfort because of a back condition. But anyone can use this sequence.

PELVIC WAVE

What has continually amazed me during my years of teaching is the unawareness so many people have regarding the pelvis. Some actually don't know where it is! I can really understand this because, on a psychological and emotional level, this is probably the most vulnerable area of the body. When most people are asked to curl (tip) up the pelvis, they look at me in confusion; then when they realize what I want them to do, they're embarrassed. It's as if the space between their waist and their thighs were encased in concrete and they have been denying its existence all their lives. To them, this area is like a no-man's-land, whose only function is to serve as the place from which you move either your upper torso or your legs. It is most interesting to me that some people have the ability to move the pelvis easily, and have the understanding of how to do it, but still won't let go of the emotions attached to it. That area represents a lot of things to a lot of people—sex, fear, exposure, parental reprimands, inhibition, power, and money. Sometimes I think it started with wearing diapers, because that's the only part of the body that's always covered when one is an infant.

The pelvis is the link between the upper and lower body. In general, its movements are secondary to those of the legs and the torso. For instance, if you want to leap up three stairs at a time, your legs would make the initial movement, and the pelvis would take over to complete it. There are no muscles solely for pelvic motion; the muscles of the legs and back control its movement. The only primary movement of the pelvis is that which originates from the pelvis itself as in the pelvic wave.

Of all my exercises, the pelvic wave is the one both men and women practice most at home, alone. When teaching new students, I discourage them from working out in front of a mirror; but in this

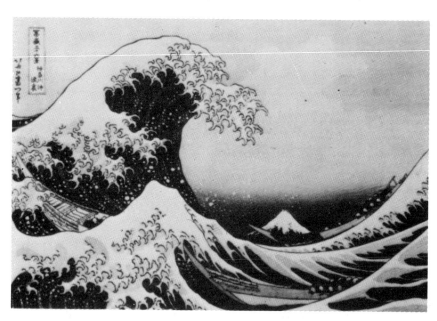

case, it helps for them to see how insignificant their fears are. I always can see a dramatic change by the second class, because they've learned it's "safe" for them to move the pelvis. Once they allow the pelvis to function as it was created to, they experience such feelings of freedom and release, and derive such benefits for the entire body, that they wonder how they could have ever deprived themselves for so many years.

Nowhere can you better feel the connection between the front and back of the body than in the pelvic wave. As soon as you curl up your pelvis, you feel relief in your lower back. And as you continue, you will be truly surprised at the elasticity of the spine and lower back muscles. You get many rewards for doing one simple motion; if you're only interested in releasing your lower back and spine, you will derive tremendous benefit by doing the pelvic wave. However, if you increase the degree of the curl-up, you will be able to strengthen your abdominal muscles, inner and front thighs, buttocks, calves, and feet. In addition, you are loosening your upper back and hip joints and learning to release the lower back even more.

When your pelvis starts to have that beautiful flow, there will be no excuse for slumping over. You will be able to curl up your pelvis with ease as you walk, stand, and sit. This will permit you to stretch your spine more comfortably to its limit and hold your head and shoulders erect.

The pelvic wave is so important that it is the one exercise I most often demonstrate on television. I invariably call on extremely strong men to place one of their hands on my lower back, the other on my lower abdominals, and then squeeze as hard as they can. (On one occasion, I recall a world-class bodybuilder gritting his teeth and breaking out in a sweat!) Then they feel and see, in living color, how strong and flexible my pelvic muscles are, how much control I have over them, and how the motions stretch my lower back. They are astonished, and confide in me (off camera, of course!) that they'd like to acquire that strength.

First you must locate your pelvis. Imagine an upside-down triangle, the two hipbones being the widest part and the pubic bone, the point. The pelvis is possibly the most important structure affecting posture, balance, and alignment. It influences whether you stand swaybacked, round-shouldered, head thrust forward, etc., and is particularly significant for lower back stability. Ordinarily, if your pelvis is in improper alignment with the rest of your body, your posture will suffer and you will most likely become unbalanced and crooked. People with swaybacks (myself included) get used to feeling the tightness in the back muscles so much that we don't even know we're tight. We become conditioned to believe that it's normal for us, and in no time many of us become prone to lower back pain. However, it's not necessary to become resigned to this discomfort, and one of the best ways to achieve the mobility the back needs to become straighter is to do the pelvic wave whenever you think of it. Until you do, it will be impossible for you to realize how drained and exhausted you become if your lower back is tensed. When you're free of tension after doing the pelvic wave, your energy and body will feel beautiful, light, and flowing—like a feather floating in the wind.

Why do I use the term *pelvic wave*? I found while on tour for *Callanetics* that everyone had his or her own interpretation of a tip-up. Eight out of ten times, people would stick their abdomen out, arching the lower back, and the pelvis was certainly not flowing. Out of my frustration to find the appropriate image, I remembered sitting on the edge of the shore and watching waves roll in. This was the exact motion I wanted, and it worked immediately to help people understand the strength and flow inherent in the movement of the pelvic wave.

An Indian general at a recent elephant polo match in the jungles of Nepal, lacking furniture, held on to the tusks of an elephant to do the pelvic wave!

PELVIC WAVE, LYING DOWN

NOTE: This exercise can be used along with floor alternatives.

When that dreadful signal, your alarm clock, announces that you have to function in the world of stress—which is enough to put any sane person into spasm—start your day the pelvic way. The following motion can waken your mind, spirit, and body because it loosens your back after sleep and helps to relieve any early-morning stiffness. You can also make it part of your warm-up exercises.

1. Lie back in bed or on floor, arms out to the side or next to body, palms down. Relax body.

2. Gently bend knees, one at a time, in triple slow motion. Place feet flat on surface a hip-width apart, toes facing forward. Permit body from top to toe to feel as though it is part of mattress or floor. Rest head on pillow if desired. Stretch back of neck.

3. Tighten buttocks muscles and slowly curl up pubic bone, as though aiming it into navel. Do not lift buttocks off surface. Hold for a count of 5, breathing normally, relaxing legs and back. While in this position, relax all other muscles, especially the abdominals. (When some people tighten the abdominals, they tense their lower back.) By all means, let go of the tension in your lower back.

4. Gently relax buttocks muscles you have tightened and slowly uncurl pelvis. Take a breather. Now allow yourself to feel the magnificent power you are discovering from letting go. Next time you curl up (pelvic wave), you can let go even more, and eventually you can be in control of your lower back. Repeat motion 3 to 5 times.

NOTE: See page 64 for instructions on how to get out of bed.

> *Once you get the feeling of the pelvic wave, you won't have to concentrate on tightening the abdominal muscles*

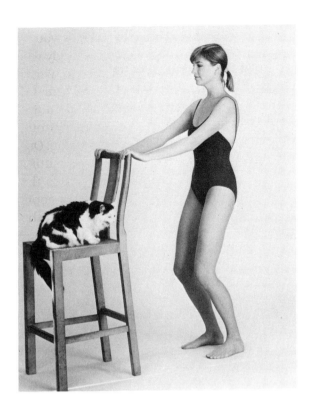

Do not hold your breath. When the directions say "Hold," continue breathing normally.

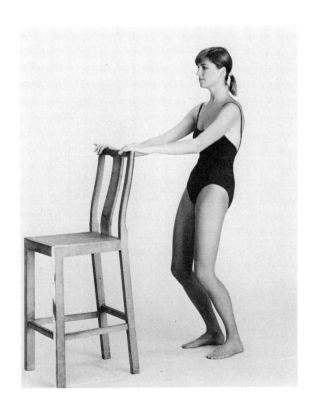

PELVIC WAVE, STANDING

Stage I

1. Stand about 1 foot from a barre, tabletop, counter, desk, back of sofa, chair, or any stable piece of furniture that you don't have to stoop to reach. Hold on to barre with arms a shoulder-width apart, elbows slightly bent. Legs are a hip-width apart, knees bent, toes facing forward. Relax body totally; do not stick buttocks out.

2. Very gently and slowly tighten buttocks muscles and in triple slow motion start curling pelvis, aiming it into navel. Hold for a count of up to 5; while holding, begin letting go of all other muscles in your body.

3. In triple slow motion, return to original position; *do not arch back*. Repeat 5 to 10 times.

NOTE: It is essential that you practice the pelvic wave in order to master it, because it is fundamental in my exercise program and in many physical activities. Visualize this tidal wave completely washing away all your discomfort and fears.

Stage II

1. Stand about 1½ feet from a barre, tabletop, counter, desk, back of sofa, chair or any stable piece of furniture that you don't have to stoop to reach. Hold on to barre with straight (yet relaxed) arms a shoulder-width apart. Legs are a hip-width apart. Bend knees more than in Stage I, toes facing forward. Relax body totally; do not stick buttocks out.

2. Very gently and slowly tighten buttocks muscles and in triple slow motion start curling pelvis, aiming it into navel even more than in Stage I. Hold for a count of 5; while holding, begin letting go of all the other muscles in your body.

3. Return to original position in triple slow motion; *do not arch back*. Repeat 7 to 15 times.

NOTE: After experiencing the first stage, you should feel more confident about relaxing your body.

(continued)

PELVIC WAVE, STANDING, continued

Stage III

NOTE: By this stage you will notice that your muscles have become more pliable and you can achieve an even greater curl. You will feel your upper back rounding, which gives you a beautiful stretch down the entire spine and across the shoulder blades. This contributes even more to loosening up the lower back. At this level you will be starting to contract the muscles surrounding the pelvis—inner, outer, and front thighs, psoas, abdominals, buttocks, calves, and feet—which, when they are sufficiently strong, begin to take the stress off the lower back. It is incredible that a tiny motion like the pelvic wave can accomplish all this and still stretch the spine and release the lower back. No wonder it is one of my students' sweetest allies!

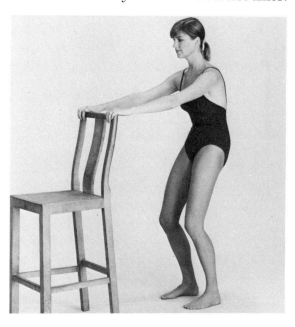

1. Stand about 1½ feet from a barre, tabletop, counter, desk, back of sofa, chair, or any stable piece of furniture that you don't have to stoop to reach. Hold on to barre with straight (yet relaxed) arms a shoulder-width apart. Legs are a hip-width apart. Bend knees and turn feet out slightly so that knees are over toes. Relax body totally; do not stick buttocks out.

2. Very gently and slowly tighten buttocks muscles and in triple slow motion start curling pelvis, aiming it into navel even more than in Stage II. Hold for a count of 8; while holding, begin letting go of all the other muscles in your body, especially your buttocks.

3. Return to original position in triple slow motion; *do not arch back.* Repeat 7 to 15 times.

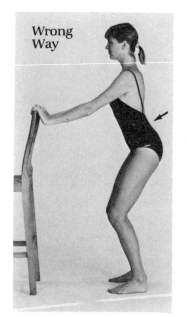

Wrong Way

NOTE: The previous exercises have prepared your muscles and spine for the following Callanetics. By standing on the balls of your feet, you will feel a more powerful contraction of the inner thighs (one of the most difficult parts of the body to tighten) and all surrounding muscles, and you can achieve almost double the flow of the pelvic wave. You will be amazed at how strong and flexible this area can become. In fact, you can keep increasing the curl to the limit of your strength. And remember, one of the payoffs is enviable posture, stature, and tighter inner thighs.

Turning the feet out and placing the heels together helps to distribute and stabilize the body's weight more effectively; it takes pressure off the knees and provides the back with a safe balance point. Most people have a tendency to arch the back. This position will make you more conscious of that habit, and give you the opportunity to correct it immediately—something you can benefit from for the rest of your life while walking, sitting, etc. Also, as this exercise has progressive stages, the position of the feet gives you more control over the motions.

PELVIC WAVE

Callanetics

1. Stand about 1½ feet from a barre, tabletop, counter, desk, back of sofa, chair or any stable piece of furniture that you don't have to stoop to reach. Hold on to barre with straight (yet relaxed) arms a shoulder-width apart. Legs are a hip-width apart. Turn feet out so that knees are over toes; bend knees. Stand on balls of feet and place heels together. Relax body totally; do not stick buttocks out.

2. Lower body 1 inch (do not let heels drop), then tighten buttocks and do pelvic wave even more than you think you can, for a count of 5; slowly release pelvic wave.

3. Still balancing on balls of feet, lower body 1 inch more, do pelvic wave for a count of 5, then slowly release. Lower body 1 inch more, hold for a count of 5, and slowly release.

4. Reverse the process, coming back up until you return to original position. Repeat complete exercise 2 more times.

NOTE: While going up and down, keep your body erect. But as you aim the pelvic wave more into the navel, your upper back automatically rounds. Permit it to round as much as possible. Soon you will feel a beautiful stretch in your upper back as well as your lower back—the entire spine.

At first you will probably be leaning over the barre and holding on to it with all your might. As your legs become stronger, you will be able to hold your back and neck erect with ease.

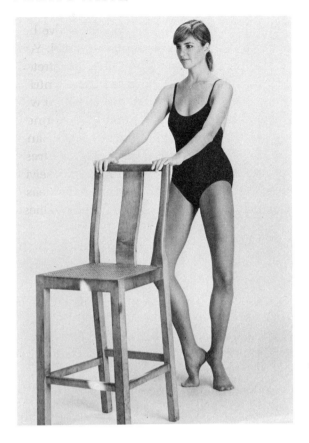

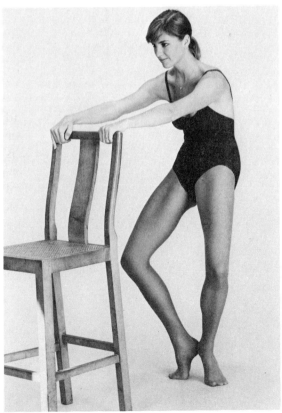

Stay on balls of feet throughout exercise

Do not stick buttocks out

NECK

I feel that the neck is the most fragile and neglected part of the body. Very few people realize this vulnerability until they suffer discomfort or severe pain. Your poor little neck muscles are always working except when you're sleeping (and even that time can be irritating, if your head is not properly supported). No wonder—the neck and the head it supports weigh at least ten pounds. It exhausts me to think that every day of my life I'm balancing a bowling ball on top of those spindly vertebrae. I only wish that when we were children in the first grade, we could have been shown an X ray of how small the cervical discs are compared to the larger discs of the spine. We probably would have taken more care to protect our delicate neck throughout our lives.

The first problem is that the structure is impractical. The neck rests at the top of the spinal column, but the head usually doesn't remain there. It's thrust out in front, because humans are frontally oriented. All their senses, especially their eyes, are facing forward, so they tend to keep their heads in that position.

The poor neck becomes a beast of burden; it does the lifting, carrying, standing, walking, running, and furthermore becomes the dumping ground for most of your tension. In the case of the neck, gravity is our worst enemy (surpassed only by the anxiety of the April 15 tax deadline). If we were left to our own unconscious inclinations, our heads would always be drooping on our chests. It's a tremendous effort to keep our heads erect, and most of our daily activities are geared to it dropping down: from professionals to laborers, almost everyone works with his head bent (except Michelangelo while he was painting the Sistine Chapel—and he probably had severe shoulder aches).

When your head drops, the ligaments at the back of your neck, shoulders, and the area between the shoulder blades become overstretched. In an effort to keep their heads erect, most people tighten the muscles in the neck, hunch the shoulders, or round them forward. As though we needed another responsibility in our lives, along comes this one: to make a really conscious effort to keep our heads erect, in the face of the wrong desks, chairs, etc. When the neck is properly aligned over the shoulders (ears in line with shoulders), its muscles don't have to strain to hold the head up. The head will automatically be balanced and relaxed on the vertebrae.

One of the primary objectives of Callanetics is to counteract this unconscious postural habit. You learn to stretch the neck, shoulders, and upper torso very delicately and gently. Your road to neck consciousness starts with this gentleness. Treat this part of your body as though it were a newborn infant who can't be thrown about recklessly, but must be stroked, loved, and respected. A gentle approach allows you to start becoming aware internally that these areas are not separate but instead are a part of you and interconnected with each other. In fact, the parts of your body are so interrelated that any difficulty with your neck or upper torso may result in lower back problems.

Often, for strengthening the neck, specific exercises involving the front neck muscles are prescribed. This is not necessary in Callanetics; the initial rounding up of the head, shoulders, and upper back in the abdominal exercises serves exactly the same function by strengthening the front neck muscles while at the same time stretching the back neck muscles, the upper back, and most of the spine.

During certain popular exercise routines, the neck can actually be strained or injured by improper motions. For instance, when I used to go to discos or when I observed aerobic dance classes, I was amazed at the abuse sustained from all the neck-thrusting. Often, we are not even aware of this until later—perhaps even years later. In my zeal to try every kind of exercise now being taught, I fell victim to this: I managed to injure my neck—something I had never done in practicing Callanetics for fifteen years. The fact was, I knew beforehand something injurious might happen, because these particular exercises employed movements that were too forceful. But I took the risk, against my better judgment.

When I spoke at a conference of over two thousand practitioners from across the country, many of them came up afterward to thank me for stressing in Callanetics the gentle manner in which neck motions should be done.

The neck exercises are first in this section because many people with back problems also tend to have problems with their necks. In fact, necks are the second most serious problem (lower back being first), possibly because of the tension that people hold there. This tension causes your muscles to constrict, which in turn reduces the blood supply to them. This can certainly cause headaches (common with neck tension) and may eventually cause serious muscle tissue deterioration. For this reason, it is essential that you know how to relax and position your neck before you continue with the rest of the program or any other program.

You can take advantage of these wonderful motions throughout the day: while watching television, speaking on the phone, standing in line, having anxiety attacks, screaming at your children, wanting to clobber your boss, etc. Now is the time to begin to learn about letting go of all the fear and stress you're holding in your neck. You will be amazed at how well it will serve you.

NOTE: Do the neck exercises only when you have time to fully concentrate on them and can do them in triple slow motion. People with swaybacks should bend the knees more to feel how even they can straighten the lower back.

NECK

Stage I

1. Stand erect with legs a hip-width apart, knees slightly bent, feet forward. Tighten buttocks and curl up pelvis (pelvic wave). Relax shoulders; don't make the common mistake of tensing them and holding them under the ears. (I always pretend Mr. Universe is standing on mine.)

2. Keeping shoulders relaxed and down, slowly lower head to the right, so that your right ear is as close as possible to your right shoulder, nose pointing straight ahead. Hold for a count of 5 to 10.

3. If you wish, gently move head no more than 1/16 inch toward shoulder in triple slow motion, 10 times.

4. Slowly return to center; stretch neck up toward ceiling, chin pulled in (not down). Repeat on other side.

   NOTE: When you lower your head to each side, you don't have to do anything but relax and just be there, because gravity is doing the work for you.

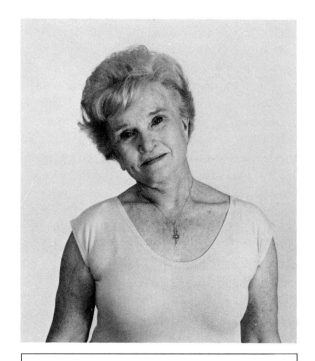

Your shoulders can always drop lower than you think they can. You must feel like you are a rag doll (either Raggedy Ann or Andy—your choice).

Stage II

1. Stand erect with legs a hip-width apart, knees slightly bent, feet forward. Tighten buttocks and curl up pelvis (pelvic wave). Relax shoulders; don't make the common mistake of tensing them and holding them under the ears.

2. Keep shoulders relaxed and down. Stretch neck up. Slowly turn head halfway between center and right shoulder. Allow gravity to pull head down so that nose is pointing toward right toe. Hold for count of 5 to 10.

3. Raise head to original position. Slowly turn head to left and repeat movement. Hold for a count of 5 to 10. Slowly return to center.

   NOTE: The more the shoulders are back, the more the stretch. Don't force your head down.

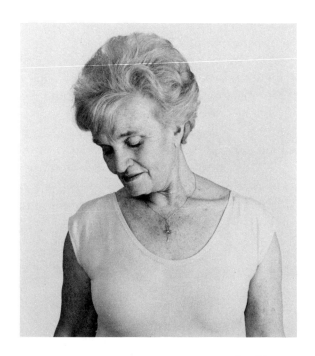

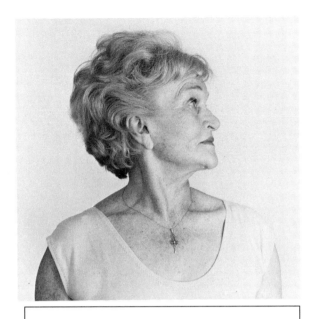

> *Whenever you stretch the neck up, remember to keep shoulders down.*

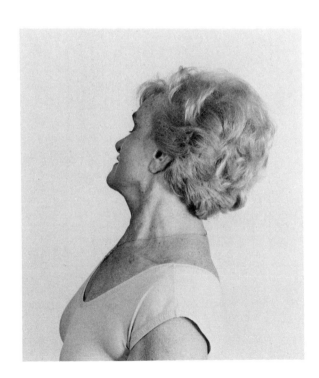

Stage III

1. Stand erect with legs a hip-width apart, knees slightly bent, feet forward. Tighten buttocks and curl up pelvis (pelvic wave). Relax shoulders; don't make the common mistake of tensing them and holding them under the ears.

2. Stretch neck up, feeling the stretch on sides and back. Keep eyes facing front, chin level, and jaw loose.

3. Turn head in triple slow motion to right and then to left in one continuous motion. Try to look over shoulders (be sure to keep shoulders facing front). Hold at each side for a count of 5 to 10. Do 5 complete motions.

Callanetics

1. Stand erect with knees slightly bent, legs a hip-width apart, feet forward. Tighten buttocks and curl up pelvis (pelvic wave). Relax shoulders.

2. In triple slow motion, stretch neck up and at the same time lower chin toward chest. Gently move chin toward right shoulder, gradually raising it a bit until nose is over middle of shoulder.

3. Stretch neck as high as possible, chin tilted up without bending head back, still keeping shoulders low (now Mr. Universe is jumping on them!). Slowly look behind right shoulder as far as possible. Stretch neck even more. Hold for a count of 5.

4. With neck still stretched, slowly rotate chin down to shoulder, then chest, moving toward left shoulder. Stretch neck as described in step 3, this time looking over left shoulder. Hold for a count of 5. Movement to *each* shoulder is counted as 1 time; repeat 6 times.

5. Slowly bring head back to center to complete exercise.

   NOTE: All of these neck exercises can be done while sitting in a chair or on floor (see pages 75, 98), whichever feels better for your lower back.

Floor Alternative

1. Lie on floor (or in bed), knees bent, feet a hip-width apart and 1 to 1½ feet from buttocks (wherever they're most comfortable). Relax head; stretch back of neck, as though trying to get it flat on floor. Chin is slightly pulled in.

2. Slowly turn head to right, completely relaxed, and allow gravity to pull it down as far as possible. Hold for a count of 5 to 10. Slowly return to center position.

3. Repeat on left side. Movement to *each* shoulder is counted as 1 time; repeat 5 times.

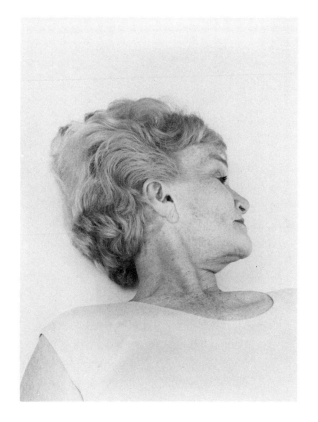

UNDERARMS

I created the following exercise in the hope that it would relieve the pain in my neck and upper back, and also help me to stand more erect. To my amazement, I discovered that it was also the most effective motion for tightening the underarm area.

When shoulders are rounded and hunched forward (as is unfortunately the case with most of us), the chest muscles are shortened and the upper back muscles are overstretched and strained. Over a period of time this poor postural habit can weaken both sets of muscles and cause the joints to stiffen. This can ultimately contribute to dowager's hump and a head that is permanently misaligned. Also, this position seriously restricts your breathing.

Some new students, when beginning the following underarm exercises, would invariably find it terribly difficult to pull their shoulders and arms back or to bring their head to a neutral position. It was as if the entire upper part of their body was fused into one rounded unit. For so many years, they had been "carrying the burden of their world" on their shoulders and necks that the motion of moving the head and shoulders back seemed impossible. The word *relax* had become foreign to them. Usually these were high-powered, successful people, overloaded with responsibility; hyperactive nervous wrecks; or victims. Yet none of us is immune to these afflictions.

I soothed and smoothed them through voice and touch, carefully and slowly. Sometimes the feeling of the muscles beginning to relax was so intense that the students would sigh out loud, at which point I would say, "Cry, scream, have a tantrum—just let whatever is coming up happen. You are releasing emotional pain, as well as muscular tightness, and it's safe for you to let go." Then they would feel more secure and could begin to work at their own pace. It was astonishing how their posture improved, even after the first hour, just by releasing the muscles between their shoulder blades.

In the following exercises, the chest muscles are stretched and elongated, with the result that the whole area loosens up and the triceps (underarms) are quickly tightened. This underarm area is often neglected in most exercise programs, yet it is the one most prone to dangling, "gooshy" flab. In addition, posture and breathing improve. You'll be thrilled with the amount of air your lungs take in and the subsequent increase in your vitality (especially helpful for smokers).

By curling the pelvis up (pelvic wave) and bending your knees, you can prevent hyperextension (arching) of the lower back and begin to bring yourself into correct postural alignment. However, you may automatically try to bring your shoulders and head forward, so be forewarned: This forward position will have to be corrected to complete the proper alignment. To do this, stretch the muscles in the back of the neck up to the sky, and pull your chin in to lessen the cervical (neck) curve. It will help you to understand this sensation if you try to balance a heavy book on your head as you stand or walk. You'll have to push up to counteract the weight of the book, and straighten your spine to keep the book from falling. During my travels, I noticed that people who regularly balanced loads on top of their heads had beautifully erect posture.

When you take your arms back to perform this exercise, you'll feel the muscles working between your shoulder blades from your neck to the middle of your back. It is quite surprising what a great effect releasing the tension in your upper back has on relaxing your lower back.

Be patient with yourself. Any poor postural condition came about over a long period of time, and you cannot expect to be totally free of it after only one or two attempts. The rewards in health, body awareness, self esteem, stature, and vitality will be well worth a small amount of your time.

UNDERARMS

Stage I

NOTE: In all of the following exercises, whenever you bring your shoulders up to your ears and then move arms to the back, allow the shoulders to relax down as low as possible.

1. Stand with feet facing forward, legs a hip-width apart. Bend knees considerably, raise shoulders to ears, tighten buttocks and curl up pelvis (pelvic wave).

2. Try to get shoulder blades to touch. Then bring shoulders down and really relax them. (Imagine that Mr. Universe is jumping on them and he's heavy!) Relax neck (chin is pulled in, not pushed forward). You should feel as though your whole spine is being stretched like a rubber band. Look straight ahead.

3. Try to straighten arms behind you without forcing them. Rotate hands so that you try to have backs of hands facing each other and thumbs aiming toward ceiling.

4. Move arms no more than ¹⁄₁₆ inch back and forth toward each other trying to touch thumbs, 10 to 15 times. Do not strain; remember to keep knees, shoulders, and neck relaxed and pelvis curled up.

5. Gently release arms in triple slow motion and return to starting position.

NOTE: At first, some people have difficulty keeping their arms straight and high, due to lack of strength and flexibility. With practice this will become easier.

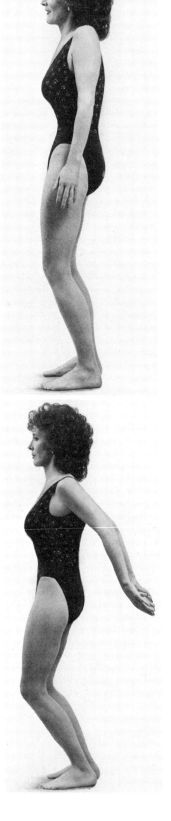

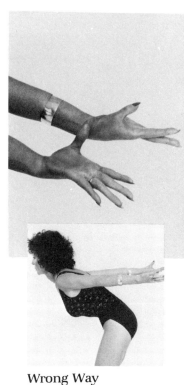

Wrong Way

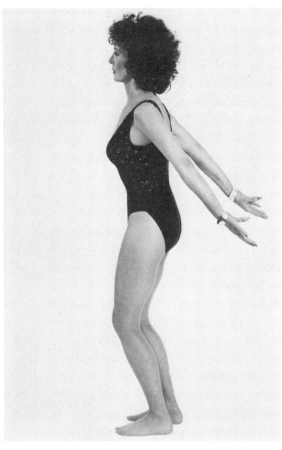

Stage II

1. Stand with feet a hip-width apart, facing forward. Bend knees less than in Stage I. Raise shoulders to ears, even more than Stage I, tighten buttocks and curl up pelvis (pelvic wave).

2. Bring shoulders back, trying to get shoulder blades to touch, then bring them down.

3. Straighten arms behind you, backs of hands facing each other and thumbs aiming toward ceiling. Stretch arms higher. (You may not be able to get your arms as close together as before.)

4. Move arms 1/16 inch back and forth toward each other, 20 to 30 times. Be careful not to arch back or stick stomach out.

5. Upon completion, gently release arms in triple slow motion and return to starting position.

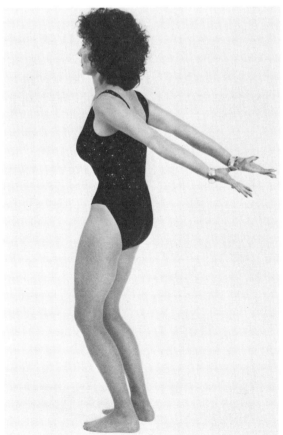

Stage III

1. Stand with feet a hip-width apart, facing forward. Bend knees less than in Stage II. Raise shoulders to ears, tighten buttocks and curl up pelvis (pelvic wave) even more than Stage II.

2. Bring shoulders back, trying to get shoulder blades to touch, and then down.

3. Straighten arms behind you, backs of hands facing each other and thumbs aiming toward ceiling. Stretch arms as high as you can, aiming for shoulder level. Be sure to maintain same posture.

4. Move arms 1/16 inch back and forth toward each other, 20 to 30 times.

5. Upon completion, gently release arms in triple slow motion and return to starting position.

> *At this stage, you might start to lean torso forward. Don't!*

(continued)

UNDERARMS, *continued*

Callanetics

1. Stand erect with feet facing forward, legs a hip-width apart. Straighten legs or bend knees slightly. Relax (do not lock) knees. Tighten buttocks and curl up pelvis (pelvic wave).

2. Stretch arms straight out to side at shoulder level; raise shoulders to ears. Slowly turn hands forward and over so that backs of hands are facing floor, palms and thumbs facing ceiling.

3. Holding head erect, slowly move straight arms to back as though trying to get backs of hands to touch (shoulders will automatically drop). Try to keep arms raised as high as possible. (Your goal is to get arms to shoulder level.)

4. Gently move arms ¼ inch back and forth as many times as possible, working up to 100. After a few motions, gravity will pull your arms down from wherever you started. Be conscious of this and keep them raised.

5. When completed, gently release arms in triple slow motion and return to starting position.

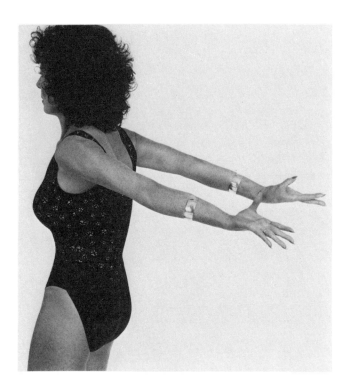

It is more important to keep your arms straight than to raise them; do not jerk them back and forth.

Be careful not to arch your back or stick your abdomen out.

Do not let shoulders and head round forward.

Be careful not to lock knees or elbows. Being conscious of not locking knees even though your legs are straight provides a wonderful opportunity to learn to relax knees.

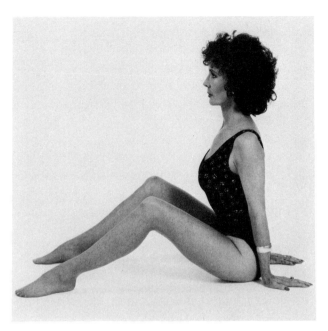

Floor Alternative

1. Sit on floor, knees bent and legs apart, feet flat on floor (feet can be turned out). Place hands on floor close to body and slightly in back. This will keep spine straight and prevent torso from collapsing. Shift hips forward to sit on "sit bones."

2. Raise shoulders to ears, then pull them back and down. Straighten arms behind you without locking elbows, backs of hands facing each other and thumbs aiming toward ceiling.

3. Lower shoulders completely in triple slow motion. Move arms ¼ inch toward each other, trying to get shoulder blades to touch, 10 times at first, then 20 times, working up to 100.

NOTE: If you find this position uncomfortable, sit cross-legged. The important point is that your spine is straight.

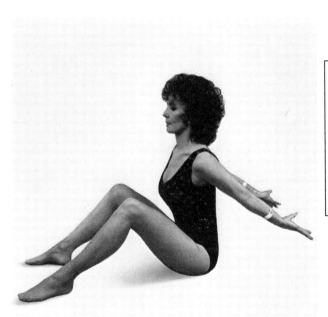

Common mistakes
- *Tensing shoulders up toward ears during motion*
- *Thrusting neck and shoulders forward; leading with head*
- *Jerking arms back and forth*
- *Locking elbows*
- *Forgetting to breathe*
- *Letting arms drop from force of gravity*

WAIST

For my condition, waist stretches are an essential part of life. There's no reason all of us can't have a smaller waist without having to resort to that dreadful "merry widow" (waist cincher), which stopped all circulation in the body and caused women in the past to faint. When I was finally able to scrutinize myself in a mirror after not having the opportunity for almost eleven years, I was horrified at what I saw: There, resting on my hipbones, were what looked like small rippled tires. And I wasn't fat; in fact it was the result of a lack of food and gravity's meanness. This really devastated me; I still carried the image in my memory of my beautifully tight dancer's body. "How does one retrieve that tight, slim, non-'gooshy' waist again?" I wondered. "Certainly not by stretching." Good heavens, was I wrong! At nearly fifty, my waist is smaller than it was when I was a teenager studying ballet.

I do the waist stretch every morning, to help straighten out my body. Waist motions stretch the muscles surrounding (or connecting to) the spine and pelvis. These help both your abdomen and back. I can feel that the stretch is elongating my back and pulling in my waist. Therefore, back sufferers derive several benefits from proper waist stretches: They can achieve a smaller waist, flatten the abdomen, and actually help their posture and back in the process.

You'll notice in all the following exercises that the torso is being supported, either by resting hands on a surface or on your body. Otherwise, if your arms are stretched up or out and not resting on something, you tend to tense your legs and lower back muscles, forcing the back to become the balance point and support for the torso. This increases the pressure placed on the lower back. When you become more confident, you can remove the support of your hand and feel the difference. In the meantime, **always make sure to support your torso with your hands**.

NOTE: In the following exercises, make sure to keep your legs no more than a hip-width apart; the farther you take your legs apart, the more strain is placed on the knee joints.

WAIST

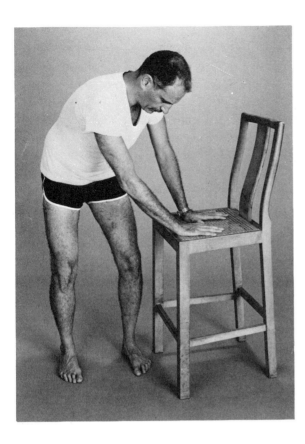

Stage I

1. Stand next to a counter or table, 6 to 12 inches away, feet facing forward, a hip-width apart, knees bent. Lean forward and allow hands to rest on surface. Bend elbows and relax neck. Hold for a count of 5 to 10.

2. With hands still resting on surface, gently move upper torso forward (toward arms) and back no more than $\frac{1}{16}$ inch, 5 to 10 times.

3. Slide or walk hands back to edge of surface. Slowly turn body to face opposite direction. Repeat on other side.

   NOTE: Be sure to keep head and shoulders relaxed. Do not hunch shoulders.

Stage II

1. Stand next to a counter or table, 6 to 12 inches away, feet facing forward a hip-width apart and 45 degrees to the right. Rest left hand on surface and bend elbow. Extend right arm straight out in front of you in same direction as feet at a height that is most comfortable. Tighten buttocks and curl up pelvis (pelvic wave). Hold for a count of 10.

2. Allow torso to move with arm forward and back no more than $\frac{1}{16}$ inch, 5 to 10 times.

3. Return right hand to surface, turn feet and body, and walk hands to other side. Repeat with left arm.

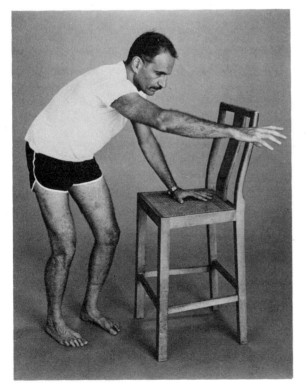

> *Be sure to keep your shoulders down. Do not strain.*

(continued)

WAIST, *continued*

Stage III

1. Stand with legs a hip-width apart, knees bent and relaxed, feet facing forward.

2. Place left hand on hip with elbow straight out to side; tighten buttocks and curl up pelvis (pelvic wave). Extend straight right arm diagonally across body or at shoulder height (wherever comfortable).

3. Slowly stretch right arm out diagonally as far as possible. Hold for count of 5 to 10; then stretch arm and upper torso forward and back no more than 1/16 inch, 10 times.

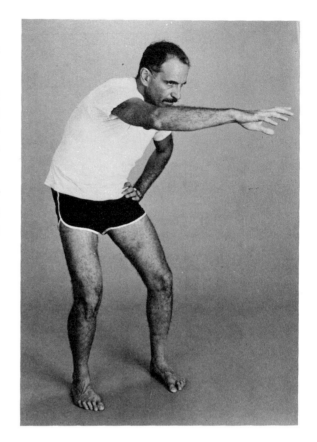

4. To reverse sides, bend knees deeply and continue stretching arm as you move to the right side. Return to upright position by curling up pelvis even more. Repeat on left side.

> *The method of coming out of this exercise eases you gently without straining the back.*

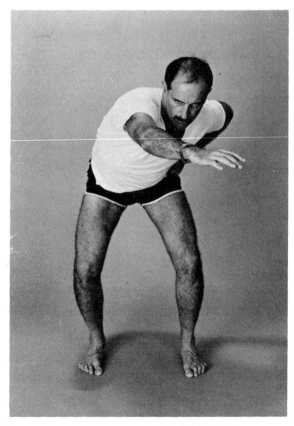

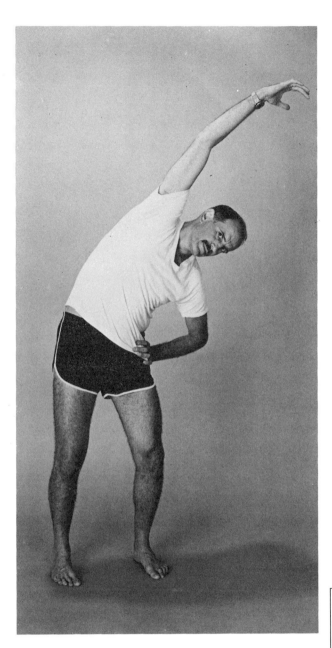

Callanetics

1. Stand with legs a hip-width apart, knees slightly bent and relaxed or legs straight but knees relaxed, feet facing forward.

2. Place left hand just below left hip to support lower back, with left elbow straight out to side. Raise right arm straight to ceiling, palm facing inward, arm even with or slightly in front of right ear. Feel the stretch from your hip to the top of your fingers. Stretch as though you were reaching two inches higher. Tighten buttocks and curl up pelvis (pelvic wave). Start reaching directly over to left side, still stretching arm up as well as over. (Imagine that upper body and arm are one unit and moving in same direction.)

3. Move ¼ inch over and back. Work up to 25 to 100 repetitions. Do not bounce or jerk.

4. To reverse sides, bend knees deeply and continue stretching arm in front of you as you move to the right side. Return to upright position by curling up pelvis even more. Repeat on left side.

5. To come out of position, bend knees more, place hands on hips or front thighs, straighten back, do pelvic wave even more, and return to standing position, one vertebra at a time.

> *The smaller the motions, the greater the stretch and the more you learn to be in control.*
>
> *The more you stretch, the more you will feel your shorts or leotard moving up with you.*

Caution: If you feel any strain in the lower back, curl up your pelvis to come out of position and return to Stage I. Remember to take responsibility for your well-being.

(continued)

WAIST, *continued*

Floor Alternative #1

1. Sit on floor, legs comfortably crossed Indian style. Rest left hand on floor close to body. Raise right arm straight up close to ear.

2. Gently stretch arm up and over to left side. Move arm and upper torso back and forth no more than ¹⁄₁₆ inch, 5 to 10 times.

3. Continue stretching arm out in front and over to right. Repeat on opposite side.

4. Bring arm back to original position and sit erect.

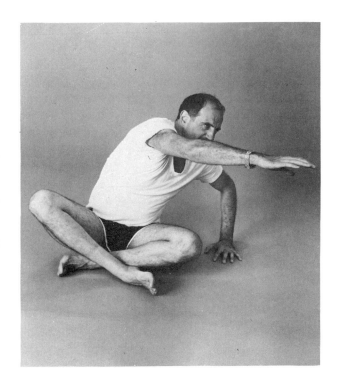

Floor Alternative #2

1. Sit on floor, knees bent, legs in front of you and feet facing forward, 2 to 2½ feet apart. Rest left hand on floor close to body. Raise right arm close to right ear.

2. Gently stretch arm up and over to left side, feeling stretch on right side. Move arm and upper torso back and forth ¹⁄₁₆ inch, 5 to 10 times.

3. Continue stretching arm out in front and over to right. Repeat on opposite side.

4. Bring arm back to original position and sit erect.

Do not round lower back. If you need to support your neck, reach arm over head and place it on opposite ear.

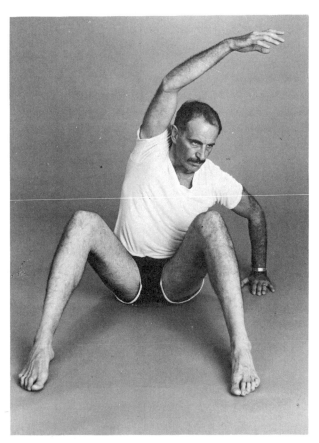

ABDOMINALS

If you teach yourself the process of being in complete control of your body, you will greatly reduce the chances of ever injuring yourself doing exercise. One way to start this is to take all stress and strain off your lower back. At the same time you'll learn to stretch the muscles of your upper back—across your shoulders and, very delicately, your neck. In a short time, you'll be able to discriminate between different muscle groups, and to isolate those you'll be stretching while contracting others. In the exercises that follow, it's as though your lower back exists but has no function. It's the feeling of just melting into the floor with the force of gravity. You are just being there. You and your lower back muscles are doing nothing.

Sit-ups are an exercise still commonly done to strengthen the abdominal muscles. My argument against sit-ups is that generally people push the muscles too hard and too fast, which means going past their limitation at that time. It has been my experience that whenever the abdominals are overused, the back takes over. In fact, traditional sit-ups use 60 to 85 percent (depending on who you ask) back muscle activity; only a portion of the abdominals are used. When people enhance their sit-ups with such items as slant boards and bars across the feet, they are making things even worse, placing undue strain on their back.

Other movements commonly used to strengthen the abdominals are "round ups," "curl-ups," or "crunches." Although these exercises employ a lighter repetitive motion than full sit-ups (you're not sitting up completely), they can still put stress on the lower back if done improperly. Whenever you begin a movement from a lying-down position and raise yourself up more than 30 degrees, you may put stress on your lower back muscles. This occurs even if the neck and shoulders are rounded. In the abdominal movements that follow, you cannot raise yourself even 15 degrees off the floor. In the rounded position I recommend, your lower back automatically sinks into the floor and has no function except to relax. Only your abdominal muscles can lift you, and they have to be extremely strong to do so. In order to strengthen them, in the beginning, the upper torso is never rounded off the floor below the shoulder blades, and the movements are very, very small. As you strengthen the abdominals and learn to stretch the upper back more, you will be able to round your upper torso even more without involving the back. Protecting the lower back while strengthening the front abdominals is an important difference between Callanetics and other abdominal routines.

Your biggest responsibility is not to rush, but instead to visualize and feel how you can relax the back more than you ever anticipated, while at the same time allowing yourself the beautiful, powerful feeling of letting go of your back. Most people doing abdominal strengthening (or any other body motions) put incredible stress on their lower back. To make it worse, they subconsciously tense the muscles of their entire body in trying to assist the abdominals.

You have probably been taught that if you don't tighten your abdominal muscles before beginning an abdominal exercise (and keep them tight for the duration of the exercise), you will get puffy abdominal muscles and a bulging abdomen. Nonsense! Muscles shorten automatically when you contract them, to the degree necessary for the activity. For instance, your arm muscles will contract with less force when you pick up a pencil than when you pick up an iron. Tension results when you place a greater force on the muscles than what is needed to do the motion. In my program, you don't have to apply excess force; simply doing the exercises will cause the muscles to contract appropriately. This is why Callanetics should always be done slowly, with great gentleness and sensitivity. Being relaxed during these exercises will prevent you from placing any pressure on the lower back, and you'll get faster results without wasting energy. In *any* form of exercise, from simple stretching to competitive sports, simply relaxing will afford you twice the stamina you would otherwise have.

While teaching Callanetics to the American Armed Forces in Europe, one of my most difficult tasks was to make the men comprehend the word *relax*. With all their experience, they had never been taught to relax their muscles. As I moved among all these highly skilled combat trainers, I gently massaged their legs or their toes and whispered, "Your body is like a feather floating in the wind. It's really okay to let go of your muscles. They should be doing nothing." You can imagine their responses at being compared to feathers! Also, these men put such effort into developing the upper part of their body and their legs that, like most men, they neglected the part in the middle. The physical therapists in the hospital told me that back-injury complaints were among the most common.

I'm surprised that the entire American forces were not lying in traction. Despite all my experience with people who misuse their back, I was shocked at the motions these soldiers made. Once they realized these were not "Tinkerbell" exercises, they desperately tried to follow everything I did. They didn't succeed—mission unaccomplished. I could see they were placing incredible pressure on their lower back while attempting the abdominal exercises. They were absolutely amazed at my strong and tight body, which was half the size of theirs—especially at my age, which was in some cases double theirs. The reason was very simple: I have trained myself to relax and contract my muscles simultaneously so that I am in control of the motions instead of the motions controlling me.

NOTE: For both preparatory exercises, it is important that you become conscious of how your back is melting into the floor. You do not have to do *anything*; gravity will do it for you.

Warning: Pregnant women in the first trimester should do *only* preparatory stretches and Stage I abdominal exercises, and these only with the permission of their obstetricians. The other stages are much too powerful to be performed during pregnancy.

ABDOMINALS #1

NOTE: In the starting position, be sure to keep a good distance between feet and buttocks. The closer the feet are to the buttocks, the harder the exercise and the more likely you are to place strain on the lower back. Also, you are not aiming to get your torso as high as possible; you are concentrating on *rounding* it.

Preparation Stretch #1

1. Lie on back, knees bent, feet flat on floor a hip-width apart, about 12 inches from buttocks. Relax neck and pull chin in.

2. Slowly raise left knee to chest (head and shoulders remain on floor) and grasp front of left leg below knee with both hands. Gently, in triple slow motion, hug leg to chest. Hold for a count of 15. Keep shoulders on floor and relaxed. Slowly return leg to original position.

3. Repeat with right leg. Hold for a count of 15.

4. Keeping right leg in position, slowly bring left leg up to chest and hug both legs with hands. Rest elbows on floor next to body. Hold for count of 15.

5. Slowly return legs (still bent) to floor one at a time.

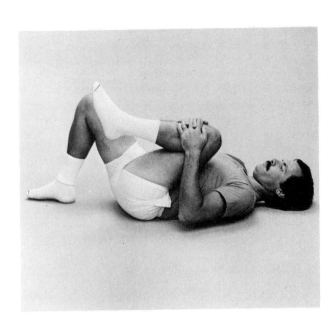

Preparation Stretch #2

NOTE: This also stretches inner thighs.

1. Lie on back, knees bent, feet flat on floor a hip-width apart, about 12 inches from buttocks. Relax neck and pull in chin.

2. Bring bent legs up to chest one at a time, a shoulder-width apart.

3. Grasp front of each leg just below the knee. Hug knees toward chest and pull both legs gently toward outside of body until you feel a stretch in inner thighs. Relax legs and feet. Keep head and shoulders on floor and relaxed. Rest elbows on floor close to body. Hold for count of 15.

4. To come out of position, place hands on outside of knees and gently push knees to center. Return legs to original position, one at a time.

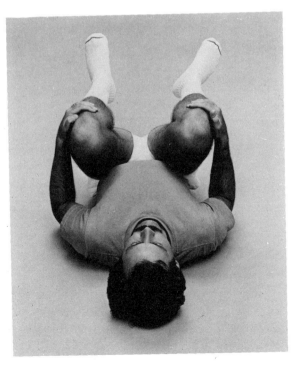

(continued)

ABDOMINALS #1, *continued*

Stage I

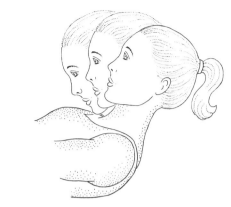

1. Lie on back, feet flat on floor, knees bent, legs a hip-width apart, at least 12 inches from buttocks. Raise legs to chest, one at a time.

2. Place hands in front of legs below knees. Gently lift head, curling upper body as though forehead were going to touch knees, nose aimed into rib cage. (Think of your upper torso as an ice-cream scoop.) Hold for count of 5.

3. *Slowly* move upper body no more than $\frac{1}{16}$ to $\frac{1}{8}$ inch forward and back, 5 times. Continuing to hold on to legs, slowly return upper body to floor, one vertebra at a time. Take a breather. Repeat 3 times.

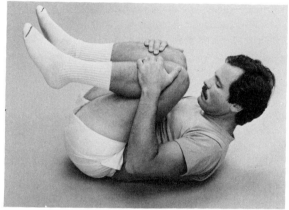

4. Slowly return legs one at a time to original starting position.

Stage II

   NOTE: Do not rush into Stage II until you feel comfortable. This is not a race. There is no deadline!

1. Lie flat on floor, knees bent, feet flat on floor a hip-width apart and about 12 inches from buttocks. Keep head on floor, grasp inner thighs, then extend elbows out to side.

2. Still grasping inner thighs, gently curl head and shoulders off floor and round upper torso toward front thighs. As you breathe naturally, hold for a count of 5. Still holding on, move upper body forward and back slowly no more than $\frac{1}{16}$ inch, 10 times.

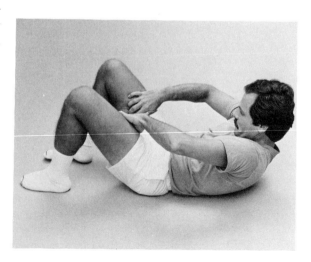

3. Return torso to floor, one vertebra at a time. Repeat entire exercise, working up to 4 times.

Common Mistakes:

1. Lifting head up first, instead of rounding head and shoulders off the floor as a unit.

2. Moving head by itself forward and back.

3. Forcibly tightening abdominal and buttocks muscles.

4. Forgetting to relax entire body.

Your arms are long enough to grasp your inner thighs without raising your head.

Variation #1

This exercise is designed for people who need more support for their neck. By using a pillow, less effort is needed to perform the abdominal exercise. You can substitute other pillows, but you must shape a wedge to be effective.

1. Position yourself on a triangular (wedge) pillow (see page 186) so that your upper back and head are comfortably supported. (Make sure that your back is not arched.) Bend knees, keep feet flat on floor a hip-width apart and about 1 to 1½ feet from buttocks.

2. Grasp hold of inner thighs, elbows out to side. Slowly round up head, neck, and upper torso, nose aimed toward rib cage.

3. Continually holding on to legs, *slowly* move upper body no more than ⅟₁₆ to ⅛ inch forward and back, 5 times. Slowly return upper body to floor, one vertebra at a time. Take a breather. Repeat 3 more times.

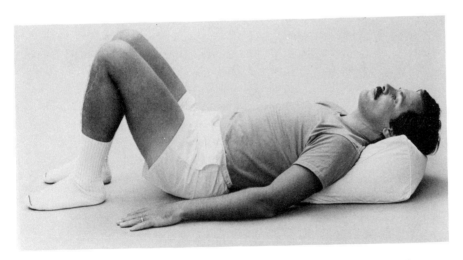

Variation #2

Any of the following abdominal exercises may be done by cradling head with hands, making sure elbows are aiming out to the side. (If elbows are facing forward, you will be stretching your neck muscles too much.) Cradling your head will help support the neck and avoid any tension there. You will not be able to round head up much; that will happen when upper back is more stretched.

(continued)

ABDOMINALS #1, *continued*

Stage III

1. Lie flat on floor, knees bent, feet flat on floor a hip-width apart, about 12 inches from buttocks. Grasp your outer or inner thighs gently, then extend elbows out to side.

2. Still holding on with your hands, gently round head and upper body toward chest as in Stage I. Release hands and straighten arms out alongside bent legs. Move upper body slowly no more than $\frac{1}{16}$ to $\frac{1}{8}$ inch forward and back, 15 times. (If you feel strong enough, do more.)

3. To come out of this exercise, slowly lower torso to floor, one vertebra at a time.

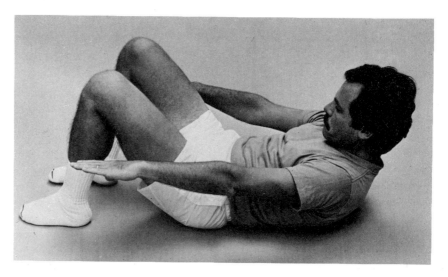

If you feel a twitching sensation through your body, that is a signal that your muscles are tiring and you are starting to use your lower back muscles for assistance. Take this as an opportunity to let go, or return your torso to the floor, one vertebra at a time, and take a breather. You will probably not be able to raise your upper body as high as in Stage II because you are no longer holding on to your thighs.

Also in the beginning you may feel the sensation in the area below your chest only and think that you are not using the abdominals. However, the more you stretch between the shoulder blades, the more you can round your back. This will work the abdominals deeper and protect your lower back. Then you will begin to feel the sensation in the lower abdominals.

NOTE: At this stage, you may have a tendency to make the following mistakes:

- tightening buttocks
- forcibly holding in abdominals
- moving entire body back and forth
- tensing or jerking body

Callanetics

This is the final touch in beginning to build incredible abdominal strength and guard against excess strain on the back to do the work. Your body should now start to feel as weightless as a feather floating on the wind. At this level your upper torso should be more rounded, your nose closer to the rib cage and the lower back, legs and feet completely relaxed.

1. Lie on floor, knees bent, feet flat on floor a hip-width apart about 12 inches from buttocks.

2. Keeping head on floor, grab hold (for dear life—not gently!) of inner thighs, elbows out to side of body as far as possible.

3. Aim elbows toward ceiling in order to feel stretch between shoulder blades. When elbows have stretched out and up as far as possible, gently round head and shoulders off floor, curling upper torso even more and aiming nose into rib cage. Still holding inner thighs, continue to stretch across shoulder blades even further than Stage III, by taking elbows out and then up to ceiling as much as possible.

4. Release hands and extend arms straight in front to outside of legs about 6 to 12 inches off the floor.

5. Gently move upper torso ¼ to ½ inch forward and back as many times as is comfortable. Return to floor in triple slow motion, one vertebra at a time. You can take a breather at any point. To continue, return to original starting position—make sure head, shoulders, and upper torso work as a unit.

NOTE: This exercise not only teaches you to protect your back while at the same time making the abdomen smaller and stronger; it also stretches your spine, alleviating stiffness in the entire back and neck, which contributes greatly to better posture. Do only what you're capable of doing—no more, no less. In my Callanetics classes, people with no back problems start with 20 to 100 times (not all at one go!) under my supervision.

Variation: Do this exercise with legs resting on chair, bed, or sofa.

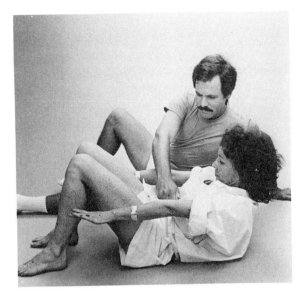

Caution: You should feel a sensation (contraction) in your abdominal muscles only—anywhere from just under the bust to just above the pubic bone. You will probably also feel a sensation across your shoulder blades, upper back, and neck, which means you are loosening them. If you feel any strain or discomfort in your lower back, stop and return to floor extremely slowly, one vertebra at a time, and go back to any of the previous abdominal stages until you feel confident. *Remember, the more you curl your upper torso, the less likely you are to place any strain on your lower back.*

Don't be sloppy by lifting your head first. When you do that, there is a tendency to pull up the entire torso using the lower back muscles instead of the correct way, which is to round the upper torso only.

The starting position is most important because it is your purpose to avoid ever letting the back take over in any movement. If you feel as though you're starting to tense your lower back, buttocks, or abdominal muscles, shift your body back and forth on the floor; just lift your feet about 1 to 3 inches off the floor and feel the difference. This position will make you aware of these common mistakes. Also, don't jerk your neck or move your arms and hands back and forth.

(continued)

ABDOMINALS #1, *continued*

Variation #3

1. Lie on back in front of a chair, bend knees, and lift legs to rest on seat. (If possible, let buttocks go between legs of chair; it will protect your back more.) You can place your hands on inner or outer thighs, or cradle head, whichever is most comfortable.

2. Lift head and shoulders, rounding into rib cage so that nose is aiming toward chest. Hold for count of 10. Move upper torso, still rounded, 1/16 inch up and down, 10 times. When you are stronger, increase to 20 times or as many as possible.

3. Lower upper body to floor in triple slow motion, one vertebra at a time. Lower legs last.

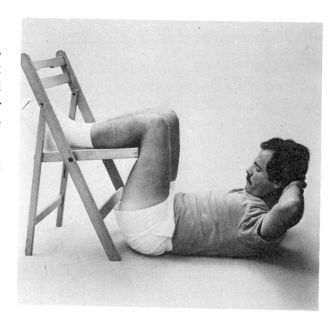

Variation #4

1. Lie flat on floor, knees bent, feet flat on floor a hip-width apart and about 12 inches from buttocks. Grasp inner thighs and extend elbows out to side.

2. Rounding upper torso and aiming nose toward chest as in Callanetics, release hands and gently separate knees. Stretch arms straight out in front between knees. Slowly move upper body no more than 1/16 inch forward and back, 10 times. Take a breather and repeat 4 times.

3. Return torso to floor, one vertebra at a time.

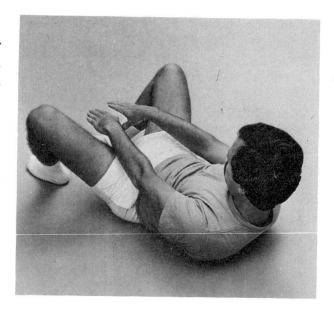

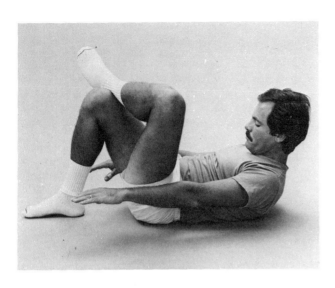

Variation #5

1. Lie flat on floor, knees bent, feet flat on floor a hip-width apart and about 12 inches from buttocks. Rest hands on floor next to body.

2. Cross left leg over right leg and rest ankle just above right knee; keep left knee bent. Rounding upper torso as in Stage II, lift arms up, 1 to 2 inches off floor. Move upper body slowly no more than 1/16 inch forward and back, 10 times. Take a breather and repeat 4 times.

3. Return torso to floor, one vertebra at a time.

Variation #6

This is included because many people like to vary abdominal exercises and this one gives the internal and external oblique muscles, which run diagonally from ribs to pubic bone, an added workout.

1. Starting position is same as in other abdominal exercises (both feet on floor, knees bent). After rounding up as in Callanetics, straighten arms diagonally to left and aim torso diagonally to left. Hold position to count of 10.

2. If you feel strong enough, move torso 1/16 inch forward and back in this diagonal direction, 5 to 10 times. Take a breather by returning torso to floor, one vertebra at a time. Repeat 3 times.

3. Repeat on other side.

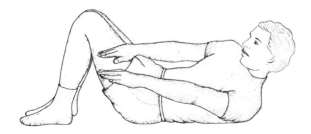

ABDOMINALS #2

Stage I

1. Lie on floor, knees bent, feet flat on floor a hip-width apart and about 12 inches from buttocks.

2. With knee still bent, lift left leg until parallel to floor. Grasp back of left thigh below knee with both hands, elbows off floor and out to side as far as possible.

3. Slowly round head and shoulders off floor, aiming nose toward chest. Stretch elbows out to side even further. Hold for a count of 5 to 10.

4. Still holding on to leg, gently move torso $\frac{1}{16}$ to $\frac{1}{8}$ inch toward knee and back, 5 times. Slowly return torso to floor, one vertebra at a time. Take a breather. Repeat 3 times.

5. Repeat with right leg.

6. Return to original position.

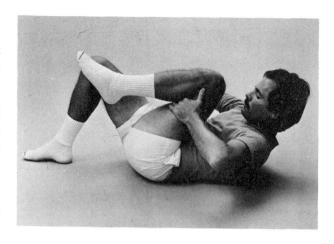

Be sure to feel a good stretch between your shoulder blades by taking elbows out to sides as far as possible. This allows you to curl the torso more into the rib cage, which in turn contracts the abdominal muscles even more. By doing this, you will become aware more quickly of when you are putting pressure on your lower back.

Stage II

1. Lie on floor, knees bent, feet flat on floor a hip-width apart and about 12 inches from buttocks.

2. With knee still bent, lift left leg until it is straighter than in Stage I and about two to two and a half feet higher than right knee. Grasp back of left thigh below knee with both hands, elbows off floor and out to side as far as possible.

3. In triple slow motion, round head and shoulders off floor, aiming nose toward left knee. Stretch elbows out to side even further. Hold for count of 20.

4. Still grasping left leg, gently move upper torso $\frac{1}{16}$ to $\frac{1}{8}$ inch toward left knee and back, 5 times. Slowly return torso to floor, one vertebra at a time. Take a breather. Repeat 5 times.

5. Repeat with right leg.

6. Return upper torso to original position, one vertebra at a time.

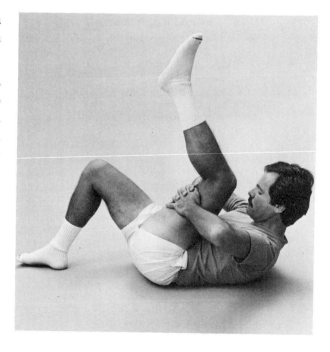

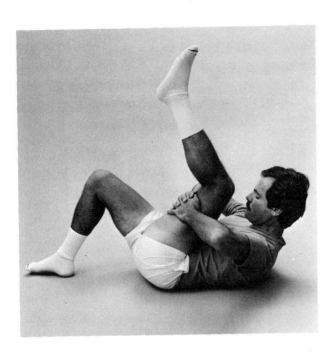

Stage III

1. Lie on floor, knees bent, feet flat on floor a hip-width apart, about 12 inches from buttocks.

2. Raise left leg even higher than in Stage II and perpendicular to body, and aim toes toward ceiling. Do not force leg to be straight. Relax leg and toes.

3. Grasp left leg in back of thigh below knee with both hands and move elbows out to side as far as possible.

4. While still holding on, slowly round head and upper torso with nose aiming toward left knee. Release arms so they are straight out at sides, about 12 inches off floor, palms down; or continue to hold legs if abdominals are not strong enough.

5. Slowly move upper torso ⅛ to ¼ inch toward left knee and back, 20 to 50 times.

6. Return torso to floor, in triple slow motion, one vertebra at a time. Bend knee and slowly lower foot to floor. Repeat with right leg.

   NOTE: Holding the leg behind the thigh will enable you to be conscious of how much the muscles between the shoulder blades are stretching. This upper back stretch is most important for people with upper and lower back problems because the more the upper back and spine are stretched, the more you can round the back, making the abdominals work more deeply and thereby becoming stronger. This helps to support the back.

(continued)

ABDOMINALS #2, *continued*

Callanetics

NOTE: Do not do this exercise until you have mastered Abdominals #1: Callanetics. Do not wear shoes until you are stronger, as they add too much weight.

In the following exercise, keep the toes of the raised leg pointed but relaxed. Until your abdominal muscles get stronger, do not attempt to lower the raised leg toward the floor; the closer the raised leg is moved to the floor, the more the muscles will contract, and that will place pressure on your lower back. If the abdominal muscles are not strong enough to hold this position, you can continue holding on with your hands throughout the exercise, making sure your elbows are out in order to stretch the area between the shoulder blades even more. Do not bring the raised leg too close to your face, either; it will prevent you from loosening the area between the shoulder blades, which in turn will prevent you from rounding properly. Remember: *Keep your leg up and upper torso totally rounded.* Be sure to totally relax and release any tension in your lower back.

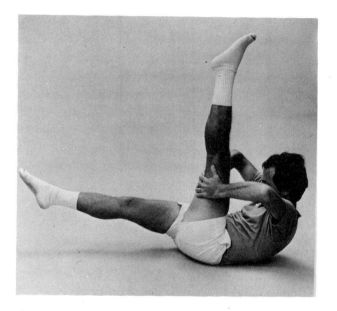

1. Lie on floor, knees bent, feet flat on floor a hip-width apart about 12 inches from buttocks.

2. Raise left leg straight up, perpendicular to body, and aim toes toward ceiling. Relax leg and toes.

3. Grasp left leg in back of thigh below knee with both hands and aim elbows out to side as far as possible. Then aim elbows up as high as possible. At this stage they should be pointed toward ceiling.

4. While still holding on, slowly round head and upper torso with nose aiming toward rib cage. Gently move right leg straight out and rest on floor; or raise straight leg 3 to 6 inches off floor (or leave it bent—whichever feels more comfortable for you). Release arms so they are straight out at sides, about 12 inches off floor, palms facing down.

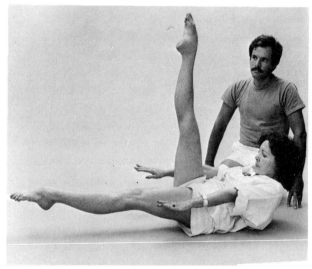

5. Slowly move upper body ¼ to ½ inch into rib cage and back 20 to 50 times.

6. Return torso to floor in triple slow motion, one vertebra at a time. Then bend raised leg and slowly lower to starting position. Repeat on opposite side.

> **Do not**
> - *Rock body back and forth on floor*
> - *Jerk head up*
> - *Aim torso toward ceiling*
> - *Move only hands or arms*

HIPS, BUTTOCKS, AND OUTER THIGHS

Three muscles make up the buttocks; the major one, gluteus maximus, is one of the strongest and largest in the body. To me, they are also the most neglected (next to the neck and underarms). When I read magazines and watch videos, I am astonished to see what the public is still being told to do to tighten their buttocks; usually, the exercises suggested employ every other muscle, but very little buttocks muscle. Even more exasperating, many of them put incredible pressure on the lower back. If I followed all the instructions that begin "This is for your buttocks," my body would probably have to be collected by an ambulance and rushed to the hospital to hang in traction for three to six weeks. Then I'd be stretched to my limit (literally!), totally bewildered, in pain, and still wondering what the heck those exercises were doing for my behind.

There is no better example of the negative effects of gravity than the human rear end. To be truly effective, a buttocks exercise should tighten the buttocks, pull it up, and reshape it to a childlike roundness resembling a peach—even in your eighties. It should seriously reduce the "saddlebags" on the outer thighs. I am still amazed when I read that the only way to achieve this is through surgery. My experience has proven, without a doubt and with documented evidence, that it's very simple to do through Callanetics. You can defy gravity and retrieve that precious little peach—at the same time you protect the back.

The following motions are a beautiful example of how this operates, because as you work the deep buttocks muscles, you are continually stretching your spine.

I craved that wonderful sensation of contracting my buttocks muscles, which was one of the joys of studying ballet. My challenge, when putting my theory into practice, was to get to the buttocks muscles without straining the back. I conjectured that if I could strengthen the muscles around the spine, they would do the work instead of my back. In my exercises, I concentrate on both the position of the body and the motion that lifts the leg to the side in order to strengthen and train the buttocks muscles to reach their fullest potential. After all, because of their large size and great strength, they should be able to do more work than just support you when you sit; their strength should be utilized to help support the lower back as well.

People have a natural tendency to arch their back when lifting a leg to the side or back in certain positions. This is especially true of those of us with lordosis (swayback). One reason for this is the misconception that other muscles are needed to move such a large weight as the leg, which can feel like two hundred pounds at first. In actuality, if you use the buttocks muscles primarily, they will do a lot of the work. The back need not be involved at all. Soon the leg will begin to feel like a feather, seemingly weightless. (The Armed Forces know that now!)

When you develop strength in your buttocks muscles, a surprising thing will happen: a long-forgotten feeling. The light, energetic step of a child will return to you; you will feel as though puppet strings are pulling your behind high into the air. You will also experience the comfort and relief of a lower back that is being supported. The difference is amazing. It will be most apparent when you climb flights of stairs, or sit for extended periods of time, or walk long distances.

Again, an important point to remember is that your body must be totally relaxed, like a rag doll. It's not the strength of the leg that is causing it to lift and move back and forward, so your legs and feet should be doing nothing; your buttocks muscles should be doing the work.

HIPS, BUTTOCKS, OUTER THIGHS

NOTE: It is perfectly all right if you can only do two movements at first. Switch sides, do as many as you can, and then return to the original side and do two more. (At this point you will probably be able to do four.)

Caution: Do not wear shoes, not even light tennis ones. They are too heavy. Do not wear ankle weights, either.

Stage I

1. Lie on left side with head resting on bent left arm. Round back and bend knees (you are almost in a U-shape). Either rest right leg behind left one on floor or place right knee on left knee.

2. Raise right leg about 1 to 2 inches. Move right knee back and forth *only* 1/16 inch 5 times. (Aim only with your knee. Make sure foot and entire body are relaxed.) Take a breather. Repeat 5 times.

3. To repeat on opposite side, gently roll over to right side, keeping knees bent. This will bring you to the correct position. Raise and move left knee back and forth as above.

   NOTE: If you are uncomfortable in any position, you can move any part of your body to facilitate the motions. Sometimes 1/16 inch makes all the difference. The more you can get into a fetal position while doing these motions, the more it will stretch the spine.

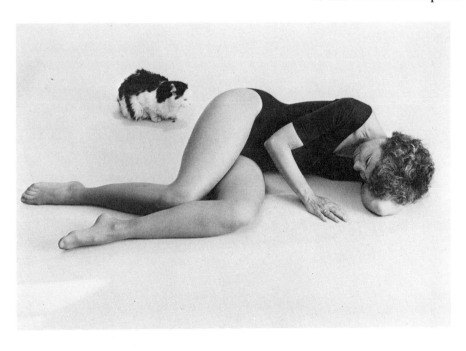

(continued)

HIPS/BUTTOCKS, continued

Stage II

1. Sit on floor on left buttock, legs bent and torso supported on left forearm. Bring left leg directly in front of you. Round back if it is more comfortable, and rest right leg on floor behind left, with bent right knee 3 to 6 inches behind left foot. Rest right hand on floor in front of you for support.

2. Lift right knee 1 to 2 inches off floor and gently move back and forth ¹⁄₁₆ inch, 10 times. Take a breather. Repeat 10 times.

3. Roll to opposite side as in Stage I, keeping knees bent. Repeat exercise.

NOTE: This is the stage where some people will want to start arching the lower back. If you feel you are starting to do it, correct yourself. This is another beautiful opportunity to learn how to be in control, instead of having the motions control you. For those who find it extremely difficult to prevent arching, tighten the buttocks and curl up the pelvis (pelvic wave) and round the back. This will stretch the spine. It will feel strange at first because you will think you do not have the coordination (you probably won't at first). Patience and practice do make perfect.

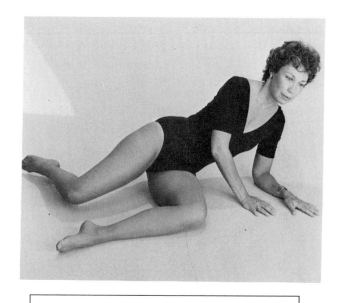

> *Common mistakes*
> * *Arching lower back*
> * *Torso thrust forward*
> * *Pushing abdomen out*
> * *Tensing legs, feet, shoulders, neck—entire body*
> * *Forgetting to breathe*
> * *Not smiling*

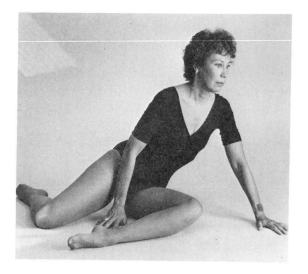

Stage III

NOTE: This is your training for the Callanetics exercise that follows.

1. Sit on floor with both knees bent, left leg in front about 1½ feet from body. Bent right leg is resting on floor, with right knee behind left foot. Torso and head are facing left and resting on straight arms on floor on either side of left leg. (If you feel that your lower back is not stretched enough, take your hands out farther until you feel a good stretch.)

2. Round back if you wish. Raise right knee 1 to 2 inches off floor and move back and forth ¹⁄₁₆ inch, working up to 20 times.

3. Walk hands back until you are sitting erect. Repeat on other side.

Variation: Follow the directions in Stage III, but use a low stool (7 to 10 inches high) to rest forearm on. Rest hands on top of each other. This is especially good for people who carry a lot of tension in their neck and shoulders; they find that resting on an elevated object relieves their pressure, and helps them to be conscious of relaxing.

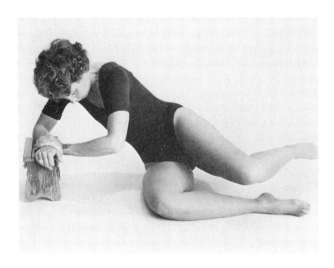

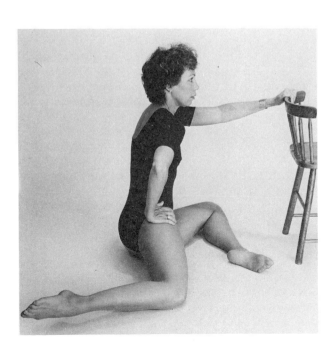

Callanetics

BIG NOTE: If the buttocks muscles are not strong enough to support this motion, or you are leaning forward or arching your back, then lean over directly to the opposite side of the moving leg as far as you wish, making sure the lower back is always stretched. If, after all this, you feel you are still arching your back, tighten your buttocks and curl pelvis up (pelvic wave). If this is too difficult, simply round the top of the back. The right knee might move a little forward, which is perfectly all right. If you feel awkward, remember that you are waking up and using muscles which have been sleeping most of your life.

1. Sit on left buttock in front of counter, sofa, table, or other stable piece of furniture, left leg resting on floor in front, knee bent and heel 8 to 10 inches away from midline of body. Right leg is out to side, knee bent and even with right hip (if this is too difficult, bring right knee forward a bit); toes are pointing back and relaxed. Left hand is firmly holding on to edge of counter and right hand is on right hip.

2. Roll right hip forward, pushing it with right hand, so that both hips are even with each other and facing forward. (Foot should come off floor; if it doesn't move, bring it up with your right hand.)

3. Place right hand on edge of object. Lift right knee, keeping even with right hip, about 1 to 3 inches off floor. Hold foot up and move right knee ¼ to ½ inch back and forth. Do 20, working up to 100 times.

4. Reverse and repeat on other side.

STRETCHES

Whereas any other young girl might dream of being the maiden waiting to be rescued by her prince, I, as a child, watching medieval adventure films, would wish to be the villain who got stretched out on the rack. I was imagining how wonderful it would feel for my spine to be completely stretched.

Most people prefer stretching muscles to contracting them, because they feel it's more pleasurable. But you can't have one without the other—contracting and stretching are essential to each other and to your body. It's like saying your teeth are more important than your gums, or vice versa.

Stretching gives you a wonderful opportunity, not only to lengthen your muscles, tendons, and ligaments, but to give vent to all the emotions that make you tense and interfere with relaxation.

You can bring a lot of your suppressed emotions to the surface and then release them like a precious bird set free from its cage (your body). Because good health begins with letting go of all negativity, this is your time to begin healing yourself. Letting go allows your body, mind, and spirit to relax.

Relaxation is one of the great benefits you get from stretching; and conversely, stretching helps you to relax. But during fifteen years of teaching, I have found that this is easy to say and difficult to do. You would think that all you have to say is, "Relax," and students' bodies become like rag dolls. But invariably, when I tell new students to relax, they immediately tense up in what they are convinced is "relaxation." From the pointing of toes to the tightening of jaws, you would think they were lying in wait for their turn in front of the firing squad.

Stretching is not second nature to most people. Those of you who are used to thrusting and jerking your bodies around, as is common in aerobic dancing, must learn how to approach stretching with delicacy. One of the main objectives of any responsible exercise program is for you to be in control and avoid injury, while at the same time protecting and releasing your back. So it is essential to understand the use of the tiny, smooth, and gentle motions: the hallmark of Callanetics.

The following exercises have been chosen from some of my regular one-hour program to help stretch all the muscles that might have been contracted during the course of this program, or those that need stretching for back stability and relief. Remember: Stretching alone does not build muscle strength.

HAMSTRING STRETCH

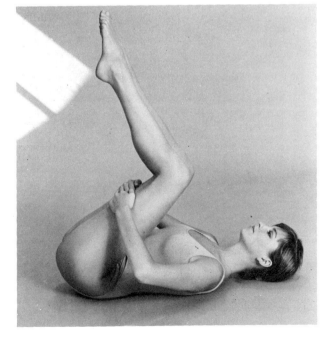

Stage I

Note: If you have sciatica, this stretch may be used to substitute for Hamstring Stretches #3 and #4 on page 41.

1. Lie on back, knees bent and feet flat on floor a hip-width apart, about 12 inches from buttocks. Arms are straight at side of body.

2. Slowly bring right knee toward chest, relaxing foot. Grasp right leg in back of thigh with both hands, straighten leg as much as possible (without forcing), and gently move it toward head, until you feel a stretch in the hamstrings. Hold for count of 10 to 15. If you wish, after a count of 10, move it back and forth no more than 1/16 inch, 5 to 10 times.

3. Slowly bring leg back to starting position. Repeat with other leg. Do 3 sets.

Stage II

1. Lie on back, knees bent and feet flat on floor a hip-width apart, about 12 inches from buttocks. Arms are straight at side of body.

2. Bring knees toward chest one at a time. Relax feet. Grasp both legs in back of calves or thighs. Straighten legs as much as possible (without forcing) and gently move them toward head, until you feel stretch in hamstrings. Hold for count of 10 to 15. If you wish, after a count of 10, move knees back and forth toward head no more than 1/16 inch, 5 to 10 times.

3. Return legs one at a time to starting position and repeat. Do 3 sets.

NOTE: Eventually you may be able to straighten your legs in Stages II, III, and Callanetics—but don't force them.

(continued)

HAMSTRING STRETCH, continued

Stage III

1. Lie on back, knees bent and feet flat on floor a hip-width apart, about 12 inches from buttocks. Arms are straight at side of body.

2. Bring knees toward chest one at a time. Grasp both legs in back of calves or thighs. Bring legs up toward ceiling as far as you can without forcing. Flex feet toward head. When legs are stretched enough, grasp toes one foot at a time and try to straighten legs even more. Hold for count of 10 to 20. After 3 times, while still grasping feet, try to straighten legs, moving no more than ¹⁄₁₆ inch back and forth.

3. Return knees to chest and cross right ankle over left ankle for a breather between sets. Do 3 sets.

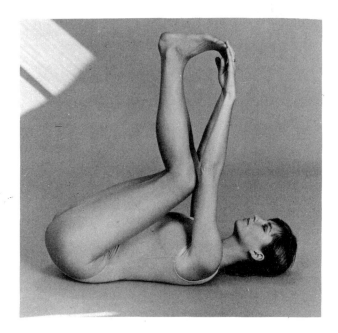

Callanetics

1. Lie on back, knees bent and feet flat on floor a hip-width apart, about 12 inches from buttocks. Arms are straight at side of body.

2. Bring bent right knee as close as possible toward head. Grasp right leg in back of calf or thigh; extend elbows to side. Raise right leg toward ceiling and straighten as much as possible. Gently bring leg toward head without forcing.

3. When you can do it with ease, slide left leg out straight to rest on floor, if possible. Hold for count of 10 to 15. If you wish, after a count of 10, move right leg no more than ¹⁄₁₆ inch back and forth, 5 to 10 times.

4. Bend left leg and place foot on floor, about 12 inches from buttocks. Release arms and bend right leg to return to starting position. Repeat on other side. Do 3 sets.

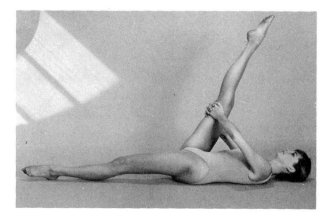

NOTE: Extending elbows to the outside gives you an opportunity to stretch the area between the shoulder blades and neck. By stretching one leg out straight on floor, you get an excellent stretch in the front of your thighs and your psoas, which is a difficult muscle to get to. When sufficiently stretched, most people will be able to straighten both legs easily. If you flex the toes of the raised foot toward your face, you will also get a lovely stretch in the calf. By bringing one leg up before straightening the other, you get an automatic pelvic wave, and consequently protect your lower back. But if you straighten the leg on the floor first, your lower back is vulnerable, unless you are naturally stretched and can do this with ease.

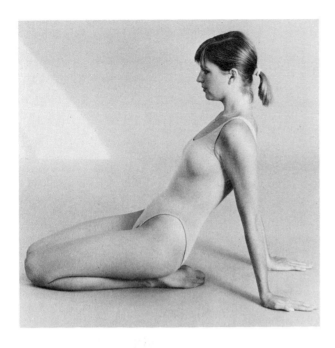

FRONT THIGH STRETCH

NOTE: Even though the following exercise might appear to put pressure on the knees, my students and I have had the opposite experience; it actually strengthens the knees because we do not maintain the sitting position for any length of time. When you raise off the heels, you release pressure on the knees.

1. Sitting on heels, with knees together or slightly apart, place palms on floor in back of your body for support. Still sitting on heels, tighten buttocks and curl up pelvis (pelvic wave).

2. After you have done this enough to feel the stretch in the front of your thighs, curl up pelvis and lift buttocks no more than 1 inch off heels at first. Try to increase pelvic wave even more. Be sure to relax your neck; do not arch back. Hold for a count of 10 to 15. Move up and down ⅛ inch 10 times.

3. Release buttocks and gently return to sitting on heels.

NOTE: If you need to, place a folded towel or other light padding under knees and feet.

For men: If you cannot sit on heels, try sitting on toes, with heels off floor, or turning feet in and sitting on them.

> *Common Mistakes:*
> * *Hyperextending neck (allowing head to drop back)*
> * *Hyperextending back (arching back)*
> * *Hunching shoulders*
> * *Tensing body*
>
> *When you feel more stretched, you may lift yourself, continuing the pelvic wave, as high as you can without arching your back.*

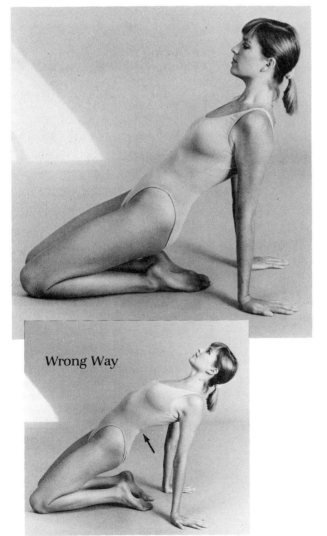

Wrong Way

FRONT THIGH STRETCH, continued

Alternative #1

NOTE: This is for people who may have trouble sitting on their heels or resting on their arms in back.

1. Lie on floor on left side; bend both knees and left elbow. Rest head on left forearm.

2. Raise right foot no more than 12 inches off floor; bring behind you and grasp with right hand. Pull lower leg behind you until you feel a stretch in front thigh (but don't bring foot to buttocks). Now do pelvic wave—the more you do it, the greater the stretch. Hold for a count of 15 to 20. Move leg back and forth ⅛ inch 5 times.

3. Reverse and repeat on other side.

Round upper back to take advantage of stretching upper torso.

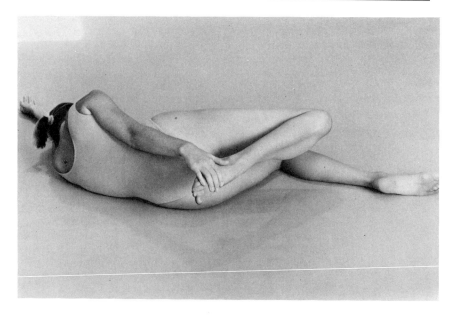

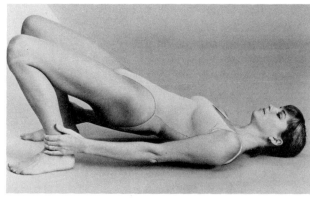

Alternative #2

1. Lie flat on floor, knees bent a hip-width apart, about 12 inches from buttocks.

2. Grasp both ankles gently with hands, curl up pelvis (pelvic wave), and lift buttocks 1 to 3 inches off floor. Hold for a count of 10 to 15. Then move up and down ⅛ inch 5 times.

Do not *arch back; stick out abdomen*

COMPLETE BACK STRETCH

This is my favorite stretch and the one that helped to align my hips. I take advantage of it whenever I can, especially on waking and going to sleep.

1. Lie on floor, knees bent, feet on floor a hip-width apart, 1 to 1½ feet from buttocks. Arms are out at shoulder level, elbows bent at right angles, backs of hands resting on floor. Stretch muscles at back of neck as though you were going to flatten them on floor.

2. Bend right knee toward chest. Straighten left leg on floor (or if too difficult, keep it bent while on floor) and bring bent right knee over left leg. Allow gravity to bring right knee as close to floor as possible. If your toes can touch the floor, let them. If not, just keep right leg elevated and relaxed. The goal is eventually to have the entire bent leg rest on floor. Make sure right shoulder and elbow remain on floor; it is more important for the stretch in the lower back to have the shoulders on the floor than to bring the knee down. Hold for a count of 15 to 60; if you wish, after a count of 10, move knee toward floor and back up no more than ¹⁄₁₆ inch as many times as you can, working up to 60.

3. In triple slow motion, bring bent right knee back to center, then rest foot on floor; keep knee bent. Slide left leg up so that both knees are bent. Straighten right leg and repeat on other side.

NOTE: Also stretches buttocks.

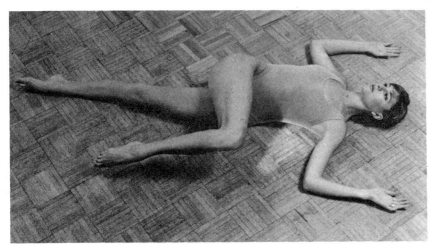

PELVIC ROTATIONS

Now that you've become familiar with the pelvic wave, you're ready to move on to pelvic rotations. The basic difference between the pelvic wave and the pelvic rotation is that the latter requires more coordination, control, greater strength.

Enormous rewards can be gained by doing pelvic rotations. You are literally lifting and holding the weight of your body against gravity with the strength of your leg muscles. In addition, you're stretching your entire spine. All the muscles controlling movement of the pelvis are getting a tremendous workout. Whereas the pelvic wave is basically a front and back motion, rotations involve moving in several directions. The increase in mobility that results from this is especially beneficial for lower back sufferers. This is the model exercise for demonstrating the concept of letting go of tension and fears associated with that area. When you've learned this, you can have maximum control over your lower back.

NOTE: If you have difficulty kneeling, you can do the following motions standing up, with knees slightly bent. It will take longer, however, to feel and *see* the rewards.

PELVIC ROTATIONS

Stage I

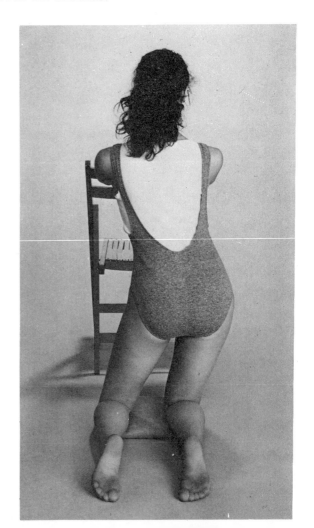

1. Kneel on thick folded towel or cushion in front of a counter, chair, table, sofa, or any other stable piece of furniture, knees hip-width apart. Hold on to edge of counter with hands. Relax body and neck.

2. Gently, in triple slow motion, move right hip to right side as far as it will go, then slowly move left hip to the left side as far as it will go, and then back to the center. Work at your own pace. Repeat 5 to 10 sets.

   NOTE: Make sure you take enough time to feel what is happening with your back. Keep entire body relaxed. Do not arch back by sticking buttocks out.

Stage II

1. Kneel on thick folded towel or cushion in front of a counter, chair, table, or sofa, or any other stable piece of furniture, knees a hip-width apart. Hold on to edge of counter with hands. Relax body and neck.

2. Gently, in triple slow motion, move right hip to right side as far as it will go; roll pelvis to the front, curling up as in pelvic wave, rounding upper back. Move left hip to left side as far as you can (the pelvic wave will naturally release). Move hips to center and then to right side again. Do complete motion 3 times; then reverse direction and repeat 3 times. If you are able to, do more.

> *Be careful not to arch back.*

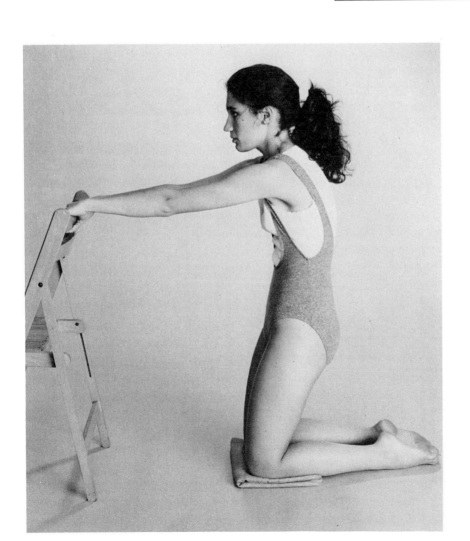

(continued)

PELVIC ROTATIONS, *continued*

Stage III: Preparation

1. Kneel on thick folded towel or cushion in front of a counter, chair, table, sofa, or any other stable piece of furniture, knees a hip-width apart. Hold on to edge of counter with hands. Back is straight.

2. In triple slow motion, lower buttocks by aiming toward heels until 6 to 8 inches off heels. Don't arch back by sticking buttocks out; keep it straight and stretched.

3. Begin to slowly come back up half the way. Return to lower position. Repeat 3 times (if you can) and work up to 10.

   NOTE: Now that your thigh muscles are strong enough to hold your body up against gravity, you are ready to move on to Stage III.

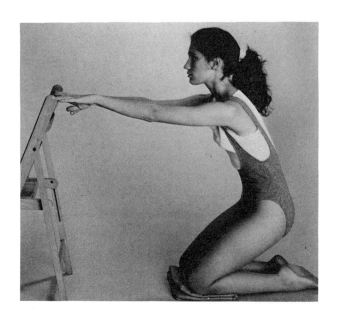

Stage III

1. Kneel on thick folded towel or cushion in front of a counter, chair, table, sofa, or any other stable piece of furniture, knees a hip-width apart. Hold on to edge of counter with hands. Back is straight.

2. In triple slow motion, lower buttocks three quarters of way toward heels. Don't arch back by sticking buttocks out.

3. Gently, in slow motion, move right hip to right side as far as it will go; then roll pelvis to front, curling up as in pelvic wave, rounding upper back. Move your left hip to left side as far as you can (the pelvic wave will naturally release). Move hips to center and then to right side again. Do 5 complete motions; then reverse direction and do 5 more. If you are able to, do more.

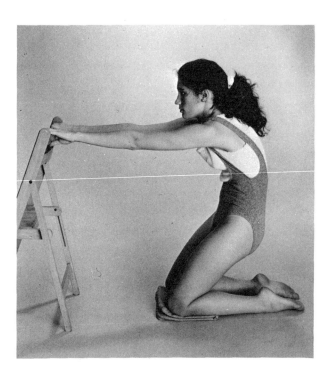

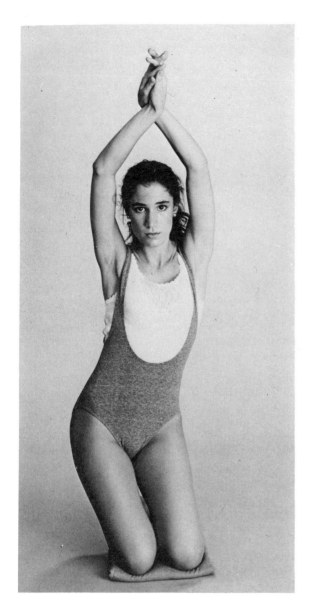

Callanetics

NOTE: Remember, you've probably never used these muscles in this manner before, so it may feel awkward at first. In fact, you will be astonished at how many muscles (that you never even knew you had) are being used. Pelvic rotations involve almost every muscle of your body. Be gentle with yourself, and be patient. Every little motion you do is building strength and stamina and making you more aware of how to be in touch with and protect your back—especially as these muscles will be taking the stress away from it.

1. Sit on your heels, back erect (lower back not arched), knees together, eyes facing front. Bring arms straight up over head, clasp hands, and try to stretch whole upper body, including neck, as if you were two inches taller. Stretch to the point where you can feel lower back stretching.

2. When you feel you can stretch no further, lift body off heels about 6 inches. Move right hip out to right side as far as you can. Move pelvis to front (which automatically will give you pelvic wave).

3. Curl up toward navel as much as possible (body will rise slightly) and slowly begin to move hips to left as far as you can. Move hips straight across to right side. Do as many as you can, working up to 10. Take a breather if you feel you need it. Reverse direction and work up to 10 on the other side. Be sure not to arch back by sticking buttocks out.

Do not try to do too much. What is important is that you don't go all the way up or down. Working in this range provides continuous contraction of the thigh muscles. Think of this as weight lifting; but instead of another force, you are using your own body, which allows for greater awareness for safety and control.

INNER THIGH SQUEEZE

One would think that after eleven years of walking around the world, I would have the tightest inner thighs in the world. Instead, at thirty-two, as I reached the end of my travels, I felt I had lost communication with my inner thighs altogether. They were just gooshy, flapping pieces of flesh hanging off my legs, swinging as I walked—utterly repulsive—and I was disgusted with them. I remembered, with sadness, how beautiful and tight my inner thighs looked when I was a young ballet student, and I prayed that there might be a way to retrieve that look (even if only 30 percent of it). That's how I came to develop this exercise. To my surprise, I found that the more I did it, not only did my inner thighs tighten tremendously, but my lower back improved as well. As I walked down the street, I was aware of such strength in that area that I could cover distances I would not have dared to walk, for fear of my back, since my return to America. That was when I realized how extremely important inner thigh strength is for support of the lower back. I couldn't disagree more with the theories that claim that all you need to help your lower back is to tighten your abdominal muscles. The body is a whole unit. We need to tighten all the muscles, especially the ones linked to the pelvic girdle, such as the inner thighs.

This exercise is so simple that at first you won't believe it could work. Yet it is so powerful that nothing else is needed to achieve that gorgeous, tight, unified look of the thighs being part of the legs—the way it was when you were a child, until disuse, misuse, and gravity took over.

Here, then, is a perfect opportunity to tighten this difficult area while taking pressure off your lower back and allowing it to relax.

P.S. Now, at almost fifty, my inner thighs are so tight and smooth that I wear shorts with pride—instead of orthopedic stockings.

INNER THIGH SQUEEZE

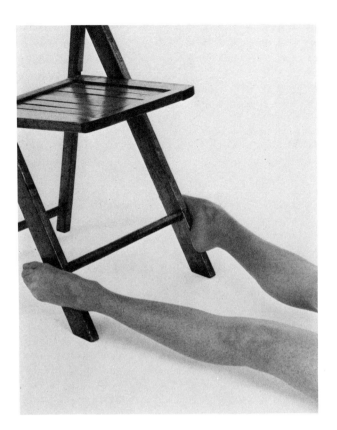

NOTE: This exercise is so easy that there are no stages. You will need a chair or a table, desk, dresser—any stable, sturdy piece of furniture with legs 1 to 3 feet apart.

1. Sit on floor in front of chair. With legs straight and knees relaxed, curl arches around legs of chair. Sit erect with top of head stretching toward ceiling, eyes front. Now, allow shoulders to slump slightly and round your lower back, keeping arms relaxed at sides (not behind you), palms resting on floor.

2. Squeeze legs of chair together as hard as you can with your feet. Make it a continuous squeeze—do not hold and relax. Squeeze for a count of 10 or longer if you can; then let go.

> *Can you imagine me telling you to slump, after my fanaticism about erect posture! The reason for this is that you will have a tendency at first to tense your lower back if you sit erect since other muscles take over to assist weaker ones. In order to prevent your lower back from straining in this motion, I would rather have you slump at first. When your inner thighs become stronger, you will automatically be able to sit erect.*

NOTE: At first you will feel the contraction on the inside of your legs above the knees. As you continue, it will move up higher, and then you will experience the enormous strength of your inner thighs. When you begin, it's perfectly all right to have your legs resting on the floor while squeezing. As you get stronger, you will be able to move them off the floor 1 to 2 inches, which makes the inner thigh muscles work more. If you are just beginning to exercise, or have just come out of spasm, you can bend the knees slightly at first. Again, as your inner thighs become stronger, you will be able to straighten your legs and sit erect with ease.

8.

Stay Away
from These

If more people were aware of which exercises to avoid and more conscious of their own limitations, a great deal of time, money, effort, and pain would be saved. I was continually shocked when my new students would bring in suggested exercise programs from their doctors: stick-figure drawings (obviously mass-produced through the Xerox machine) were meant to provide them with an "individualized" therapeutic program. It would have been a laugh if it weren't so serious. They were so "individualized" that two students, with entirely different medical problems, presented me with the *same* stick figures doing the *same* exercises. And both had the *same* doctor!

No one is more convinced of the value of exercise than I. But one can't do exercise just for the sake of doing it. Some exercises are useless and are a waste of your precious time; some require the agility of a trained athlete. All should be evaluated in terms of your own profile—ability, age, physical condition, and flexibility. I say that around thirty (even though others say forty) is the point where your age begins to matter in terms of exercise. Your age is also directly related to the amount of time it takes to get into condition and how quickly you get out of condition. I feel the average time it takes to get out of condition is 1 to 2 weeks without exercising. If you are not used to exercise, you may have to work more slowly and carefully.

As I've said before, when it comes to our bodily structure and capabilities, we are not all created equal. In fact, we should welcome the differences. Can you imagine what it would be like if we all looked and walked the same? It would resemble a fantastic futuristic world with clones coming off an assembly line every few seconds. Naturally, I would want to design the mold to make sure every unit (person) would be correctly aligned, with beautiful posture and perfectly sculptured musculature. At that point, every unit would feel so good about its body that the law would have to be changed to allow every clone to walk down the street stark naked—that's how ideal everyone would feel. There's only one thing wrong with this vision: It's utterly boring to live in a world without variety. Yet many exercises outlined in books or magazines, or demonstrated at health clubs, look like they were designed for just such a world: the same exercise for everyone.

Even worse, some popular exercises are downright dangerous and put enormous stress on the muscles, joints, and ligaments, resulting in soreness, sprains, and greater injury. The lower back is particularly vulnerable to incorrect exercising, which can both cause and aggravate chronic back problems. Due to the growing number of injuries from such activities as jogging and aerobic dancing, more attention is being paid to the dangers of certain exercises, and I'm terribly pleased about it. I hope that everyone approaches exercise with the right kind of critical eye. For instance, if I had been unaware enough to do some of those "stick-figure exercises," I would probably have ended up right back where I started—ready for a wheelchair, or at least in therapy.

Pain is a key word. If you are out of condition and start doing certain exercises, it is natural to feel some discomfort. But there are exercises that may cause you pain, regardless of your condition or how much you practice them, and you *must* pay attention to avoid these. They are probably doing something wrong to you—pushing or bending something or somewhere you shouldn't. Joints, such as those in the neck, knees, elbows, and back, are particularly susceptible. I don't care whether the movement is a contraction or a stretch; there are negative exercises in all categories.

A holdover from the old days and still, unfortunately, popular are those exercises involving bouncing, jerking, locking knees, and arching backs, which have already been proven hazardous. Sometimes a stretch, while not harmful in itself, can become so when you try to get in and out of a position.

What follows is a summary of the exercises I feel are some of the *worst*, categorized according to area of the body for which they're designed. As it is impossible to cover every exercise around, it might help to have some criteria by which to judge an exercise:

- Avoid arching your back (especially if you are swaybacked). I'm not referring to onetime tests conducted by professional therapists or doctors, or hyperextension that's part of athlete's training, or when prescribed for people who lack a natural curve. (When a person's spine is too straight, he or she may actually get relief from hyperextension.) What I object to are exercises that involve repetitive and sustained back-arching.
- When you have to lift a leg up on a surface, it's a good idea to ask yourself, "Is that too high for me at this time?" I suggest you begin by putting your leg on a low object and gradually experimenting with greater heights. Do not assist leg with your hands while lifting it because you could be forcing it beyond its capability.
- When bending over, always bend from the hips, not from the waist.

- Never lock the knees.
- Avoid bouncing, jerking, and lunging.
- Avoid any motion that puts pressure on the knees (such as twisting and squeezing knee joints), elbows, neck, and back.

HAMSTRINGS

Toe-touching (standing). This is one of the most common stretches and is often recommended for limbering up. There's a lot of controversy about this one and rightfully so. In theory, this is fine if you are sufficiently stretched, and able to do it. In practice, it's usually an entirely different story. Many people—even those who are classified as fit—have tight hamstring muscles, yet the ability to touch your toes is still used as yardstick of fitness. This is ridiculous! For some people, no amount of stretching is going to give them enough flexibility to touch their toes. So if that's their objective, they will probably overstretch, which can cause the ligaments to lose their elasticity and consequently affect joint stability. In addition, they usually lock their knees (making them more prone to injury) and bounce, thinking it will help them stretch farther. The result of all this can be torn muscles and tendons and overstretched ligaments. As I've said many times, bouncing has the opposite effect of stretching.

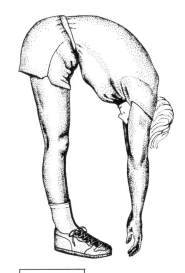

STAY AWAY

I am shocked to see people who are still jerking and bouncing with locked knees while warming up for jogging first thing after getting out of bed!

The major problem with this exercise is how it can hurt the lower back, because most people bend from the wrong place. If you want to do toe-touching correctly, you must bend from the hips. The hip joint is the place where the torso meets the leg, and is much lower than most of us realize. Many people think the hip joints are somewhere near the waist, so they bend from the waist, placing enormous pressure on the lower back, aggravating any sciatic nerve trouble, and probably not stretching the hamstrings enough to be worth all the risk.

To do a proper toe touch, release the knees (bend them even more if your hamstrings are tight); bend from the hips and lower your torso slowly, one vertebra at a time, as far as you can go *without forcing*; and gradually ease the legs straight (knees not locked) as much as you can without straining your back. When you're finished, bend your knees, tighten your buttocks and curl up your pelvis (pelvic wave), and come up very slowly, one vertebra at a time. If you want to do a really safe toe-touching exercise, sit in a chair, bend both knees, and very gently and slowly bend the torso from the hips down toward the floor (see page 77).

Toe-touching (sitting): With both legs straight out in front, this presents difficulties similar to the previous toe-touching exercise: Because the hamstring muscles do not normally stretch very much, you will probably place the work on the lower back. (This happens because the lower back is not stretched enough and the upper back is not rounded enough.) Unfortunately, this is a popular stretch to do with a partner, who stands or sits in front of you and pulls you forward. This could be dangerous because the partner can stretch you too far.

Hurdler's stretch is another common hamstring stretch. This one is done sitting on the floor with one leg straight out in front, the other leg bent back at the knee either alongside or under thigh with weight of body resting on it. This is an extreme and unnatural position for the knee and puts too much pressure on the knee joints. For this reason, it is a harmful exercise and should be avoided.

Lunges. These come in several varieties, and I don't like any of them, unless you're highly trained. One is the "Japanese split," in which you stand with both legs as far apart as possible and bend the upper body forward so that your hands touch the floor. This strains both the knees and the groin. Worse still is the next step of the "Japanese split," in which you bend one knee trying to get it to touch the floor while stretching the other leg straight out to the side—a very good way to lose your balance. The same is true when you do this lunge from a standing position, and then squat down with one knee bent and extending the other leg to the back. Another bad lunge is the one in which you rest your weight on one knee on the floor and stretch the other leg all the way out to the side or back.

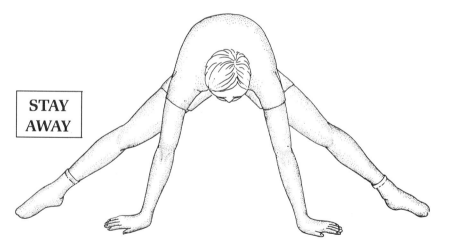

STAY AWAY

FRONT THIGHS

Deep-knee bends. If this were a "shallow" knee bend, it would be all right as a front thigh strengthener. Most deep-knee bends have you standing on your toes with knees facing forward. That's the first problem: If you squat down from this position more than 6 inches, you may be placing many times your body weight on your poor knees. Deep-knee bends, squats, duck walks, and Russian bounces stretch and endanger the ligaments of the knee, compress the kneecap, damage other joint strcutures, and interfere with your center of gravity. Duck-walking is potentially so harmful that it was the first exercise to be cited as such by the President's Council on Physical Fitness. A safer way to strengthen the thighs is to hold on to a barre, turn the knees out to the side, stand on toes, and not allow the buttocks to go lower than the knees.

Front thigh stretch. In one common front thigh stretch, you lie on your back on the floor with both knees bent, feet alongside the buttocks. When you do this, you not only strain your knees, but if you are like most people who are not stretched enough to do this, you will tend to arch your back.

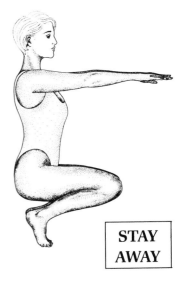

STAY AWAY

The reverse of this stretch is just as bad. In this one, you lie on your stomach, knees bent, feet on buttocks; with your arms behind you, you grasp your ankles or feet, pulling the feet and upper body toward each other, as though you were a bow. This is supposed to be a front thigh stretch, and it does stretch those muscles. But I think the real name for this position should be "destruction of the knee joint." In addition to overstretching the ligaments of the knee, lying like this can contribute to lower back strain by jamming the vertebral joints, crushing the discs, and pinching the nerves. (The safer way to do this stretch is described on pages 129–130.)

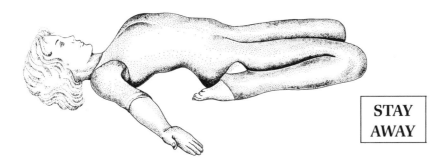

STAY AWAY

SPINE

Exercises that particularly stress the lower back are sit-ups with straight legs, double leg raises, and the swan, in which you balance on your abdomen and hold arms and legs straight up behind you, back arched—of course.

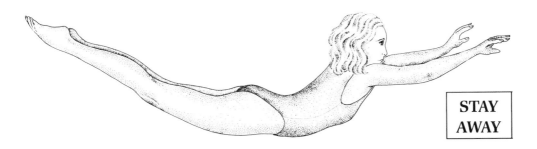

STAY AWAY

Hyperextension exercises. There are stretches and exercises that emphasize hyperextending (arching) the lower back to counteract slumping. One common example: Lie on your stomach and raise your upper torso by arching your back; the cobra position in yoga is similar to this. I believe arching the back is really harmful; there is just no safe way to do it. A certain amount of hyperextension is normal and can't be avoided in the course of everyday activities and certain sports. But persistent arching of the back can cause the spinal discs to become worn down (it puts particular strain on the fourth and fifth lumbar vertebrae), and jam joints together.

Back bends. These are best left to the acrobats. They are fraught with all kinds of risks—injuring your wrists, losing your balance, and overarching your back.

NECK AND SHOULDERS

Shoulder stand. This is called by different names, depending on who is teaching it. Also, there are variations (the plough in yoga; bicycling with legs up in the air). This exercise can feel wonderful because of the stretch in the upper back. But there are far safer ways to get the same stretch. Any exercise that has you resting your weight on the area higher than your shoulder blades is potentially harmful to the neck. It's all right to rest the weight of your torso on the area of the back ribs—the vertebrae there are much stronger—but the area above cannot stand that much weight; even if you support your torso with your hands, the position crunches the more fragile vertebrae of the neck and puts too much pressure on them. Shoulder stands also stretch the neck muscles too much and too fast.

The problem is aggravated if the stretch is performed with a rounded back. This not only stresses the neck, but compresses the upper spinal cord and chest, making breathing difficult. There seems to be some indication that some people who spend years doing yoga positions like these suffer from disintegrated cervical discs. To me, it's like a bulldozer parking on a delicate rose, that poor little fragile flower!

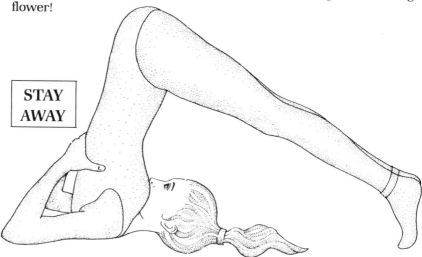

STAY
AWAY

Headstands. One correct way to do a headstand might be to have a hole in the floor for your head to rest in! In this way you could keep your head lower than your hands and take the weight off your cervical spine (neck). Certainly it's possible, with care and the right training, to do a correct headstand; but most people balance all their weight on the neck vertebrae. In addition, you could easily lose your balance, increasing the risk of injury.

Neck rolls. Many neck relaxation and stretching exercises involve turning the head in a complete circle: side, front, side, back. The danger with letting a head that weighs at least ten pounds, drop back on its own is that it puts enormous pressure on the cervical (neck) discs and can actually create misalignment of the vertebrae of the neck. Eventually, you may lose the spaces between the discs and can suffer a variety of neck pains and even numbness from pinched nerves.

Push-ups. Usually done on the floor or against a wall or a piece of furniture, this exercise is used to develop shoulders, chest, and upper arms. Women are told to bend knees with ankles crossed. My objection is that this exercise puts too much pressure on the lower back. If your upper back muscles, arms, and wrists are not strong enough, you'll end up supporting your body's weight with your lower back, and probably will arch it—especially if you are swayback.

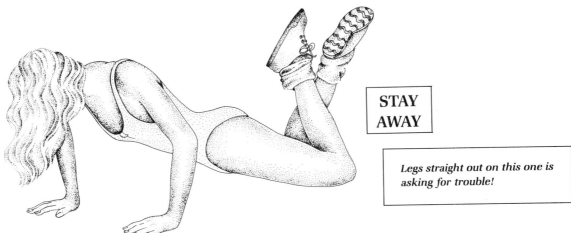

STAY AWAY

Legs straight out on this one is asking for trouble!

WAIST

Waist circles. Perhaps the most common (and sometimes the most inventively silly) waist circles have harmful consequences for the back. Whether they're circles or twists, they involve rotating the vertebrae, which can cause stress to the discs, muscles, and ligaments in the lower back. If you do them in a jerking and rapid manner, twists can result in more stress, pulled muscles, pain in the lower back, and loss of balance. The backward position of waist circles is particularly dangerous to the lower back because that area must bear the weight of the entire upper torso. They should be avoided at all costs for anyone with lower back problems. Don't feel that you're missing out—they don't do anything to pull in your waist.

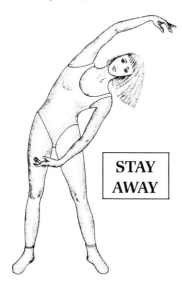

STAY
AWAY

Waist bends. The greatest danger with these exercises is that there is no support for the lower back, so it has to bear the weight of the torso; in actuality, the lower back becomes the balance point. The correct way to do this is to place your hand over the hip joint for support (a direction I notice others are copying—thank goodness!) (see pages 106–107). Another problem is that you tend to spread your legs too far apart and lock your knees. In addition, when you bend to the side (without curling up your pelvis), you'll probably arch your back, especially if you're swaybacked. And finally, because this is an exercise usually done with great ferocity (you're so eager to get your waist smaller fast), you risk pulling muscles and spraining ligaments. Using props such as towels and beach balls may place your balance in a precarious position, so in order to avoid toppling over, the tendency is to tighten the lower back—definitely not advisable.

ABDOMEN

Sit-ups. Sit-ups come in many forms and are still, unfortunately, the most popular exercises recommended for flattening the abdomen. Strong abdominal muscles are supposed to be the key to combating lower back problems, but most sit-ups achieve the opposite effect—they actually strain the back. I don't care how imaginative or inventive they are (feet hooked under bar, someone holding your feet, or on a slant board), or whether you sit, roll, or curl straight up from a lying-down position, you still put too much pressure on the back if you go any higher than 30 degrees (just below the shoulder blades) off the floor—and chances are you will go higher. It's common to do sit-ups rapidly, and this makes matters worse, because you'll probably begin to arch your back, use your hip flexors, tighten your leg muscles, balance on your coccyx, strain your neck, etc.—in other words, use muscles other than your abdominals to help raise your body. There is no question in my mind that sit-ups are an unsafe means of acquiring a firmer abdomen.

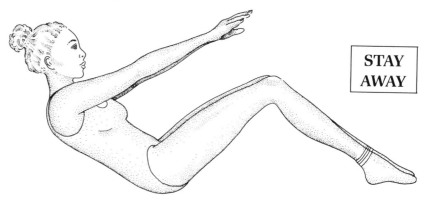

STAY
AWAY

Leg lifts. Another "tummy tightener" you can do without. Stay away from any exercise that requires you, while lying down, to raise both legs straight up or down and keep head and shoulders flat on the floor. There are many variations on this theme: leg lifts done lying down on back or side, partially seated, or even in a chair. But no matter which position you choose, this exercise definitely stresses the lower back. You're actually lifting 40 percent of your body weight! In the example shown here, you are told to keep your lower back flat on the floor, which is almost impossible for most people. So after a certain point, the abdominals become fatigued and other muscles are used to lift the legs; the hips flexors take over, the pelvis rotates forward, and the back arches.

STAY
AWAY

BUTTOCKS

Leg thrusts. Leg thrusts come in a variety of styles, but all can be recognized by the thrust of the raised leg to either the back or side while you're on all fours on the floor. These are the exercises that many fitness instructors feel are primary for tightening the buttocks muscles. (You can read in one book that they're for the legs, and in

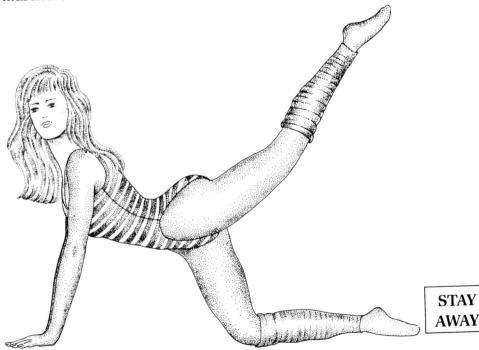

STAY
AWAY

another that they're for the hips.) Regardless of what they're intended to firm, I feel they're not as effective as they are claimed to be, and in fact are potentially harmful. I find it hard to believe that in 1988 these are still done. My main complaint is that you're required to lift the leg above the level of the hips (rather than remaining parallel to the floor). When you do this, hyperextension takes place, the pelvis rotates, and you cannot avoid arching your back. You're also in danger of falling, or at the very least of losing your balance. This exercise places excessive strain on your knees and wrists. Added to this is the rapid, jerking motion (and sometimes even weights on the ankle) of the raised leg, which can create further strain to the lower back, and assuredly increases your chances of falling (which has happened). Actually, if you do this exercise correctly (hold your leg in the lower position to avoid hyperextending), it becomes ineffective for tightening the buttocks, so why bother?

Pelvic push-up. This resembles the Bridging exercise (see page 30), which has nothing to do with tightening the buttocks! The pelvic push-up is done by lying on your back with your knees bent and feet flat on the floor, pushing against your hands and feet to lift your body off the floor as high as possible. Contracting the buttocks during this exercise is supposed to make them tight and shaped. No matter how you do it—knees apart or together, both feet on the floor or one leg straight and aiming up—it just doesn't accomplish anything, except probably to arch your back. When you push your buttocks so high in this position, you hyperextend your back, push your abdominals out and put considerable strain on your neck and shoulders; ironically, in that position, you will find it's more difficult to contract the buttocks muscles, which is the very thing that is required to tighten your behind. Try to figure that one out!

RESISTANCE EQUIPMENT

Putting pressure on your back is a common problem when working with types of resistance equipment. Most machines are not set for your specific strength and range requirements. When you're lifting such a heavy weight, you will call on your lower back for assistance if your other muscles are not strong enough. This is especially true for those exercises in which you lift both legs against a weight (to develop thigh muscles). Even doing one leg at a time is risky for the lower back.

A popular exercise using weight equipment involves raising the arms above the head while either standing or sitting, grasping a bar and then pulling it down against resistance. It develops the shoulder, chest, and upper back muscles. But it may also cause excessive strain. Most people have a tendency to arch their back as the weight increases, and probably use neck muscles to help them pull. I am also opposed to wearing weights while exercising. I feel that even the two-pound ankle weights put too much stress on the back.

9.
People Helpers

Wouldn't it be wonderful to pick up a book and learn everything you needed to know not only about the back, but about *your* back? The problem is that no such book exists, and no two practitioners, whether they're medical doctors or people engaged in body work—agree on everything.

The one common complaint that runs through all the stories I've heard people tell about their back problems is that the number of people and methods they tried was almost limitless. It seems as though most back sufferers would try anyone or any means that someone else said worked. I've known some people who have gone to as many as nine different "helpers" (doctors, masseurs, exercise people, etc.) in the course of two weeks!

Because nobody has all the answers, the decision seems to rest with you. You may be fortunate enough to find the right person or technique immediately; or you may have to shop around. The chemistry between you and the practitioner is extremely important. You must feel comfortable and secure, emotionally as well as physically, especially if the treatment involves physical contact. Sometimes you can benefit from a combination of approaches. And of course there are times to see a medical doctor.

Some reasons to see a doctor:
- *Distinct weakness in one leg or both legs*
- *Pain in back or leg(s) that is not getting better regardless of treatment or that has persisted for four weeks*
- *Fever (not associated with a cold) along with pain in back or leg(s)*
- *Loss of weight and/or pain in other parts of body*
- *Pain or swelling in joints*
- *Trouble with urination*
- *Numbness or tingling in arms, legs, fingers, or toes*

However, I feel strongly that no matter what primary care you decide on, a proper exercise program must go along with it. Choosing an exercise teacher is one of your more serious responsibilities. Even when your doctor or other practitioner has suggested exercise, the choice of which kind is still yours. Do not jump into a program because you think it's fun or fashionable. Many teachers feel that keeping the students entertained so they won't be bored and quit is most important. Safety is not an issue for them. Be careful—regardless of the fashion, it's not fun to be injured.

Look for a studio with a good reputation, teachers who have *years* of experience, some awareness of anatomy, physiology, and kinesiology, and enthusiasm for what they're doing. A good teacher knows how to pace a class and how to instruct an individual, while at the same time teaching the group. At your introductory session, ask questions, observe the class, and *walk* through the motions in the back of the room; use the rest of the time to notice if the instructor watches individual students and corrects them and if the directions are clear, detailed, and graphic (rather than shouts of trite encouragements, such as "Oh, yeah, baby, go for it!"). In order for the program to be helpful to you, make sure you are an informed consumer. One of the aims of this book is to help you do this.

Here's my favorite exercise story: In a major city, one studio found its classes growing too large for the space, so the leader (eighteen years old) took the clients (some of whom were old enough to be her parents or even grandparents) into the streets, and—mind you, in their aerobic dancing shoes—they continued their class, running and leaping on cement. While watching this "sitcom," the leader screamed, "Move it—you're going too slow." Some of the students not only found it impossible to keep up the pace, but actually sought out places to sit, and, lacking that, plopped down on the pavement, hoping to catch their breath. Meanwhile, the leader, oblivious to this, was still urging them on, not having any conception of the aging process, how it slows you down and how you must accommodate it. She probably thought menopause was a new soft drink!

Unqualified instruction is one of the main problems in the exercise business. A study of 135 aerobic dance instructors in San Diego used as its standard a certificate or degree in physical education. Only 22 percent had the educational qualifications, and 76 percent of the leaders had injuries sustained while leading (they don't teach) the class. What's more, they were ignorant of basic safety precautions. This was borne out by the fact that nearly half their students were injured at some time during their course.

Aerobic dancing and low-impact certificates can be obtained by mail order for anywhere between thirty and ninety dollars. I've received several that offered me an instructorship after a two-hour course. My favorite was a low-impact diploma for a half hour of training. With this certificate, one becomes a "qualified" teacher; over 25,000 people in the United States have this certificate, according to one ad. Unfortunately, in this case, the advertising is probably not misleading. In another scheme, just ordering tapes makes you qualified to teach—whether you watch the tape or not. There are no age or experience qualifications.

But you don't even have to invest in someone else's program. Anyone can have his or her own aerobics dance/low-impact training school with no background whatsoever. Just get pamphlets and certificates printed, pick out names from the phone book, buy the stamps, and—voilà! Instant money. This is the depths of low integrity; it's pathetic and irresponsible.

Naturally, these statements don't apply to all aerobic dancing or low-impact instructors; some of them are very conscientious.

In the final analysis, for *any* exercise program, it's up to you to learn (and feel) what's best for your condition.

The worst pitfall, though, is believing the frequently repeated "To be fit, one must accept injuries." Everyone says this—professionals as well as average exercisers and sports enthusiasts. Think about it for a moment. It bears a striking resemblance to the "no pain, no gain" mentality. Preventing injuries is very easy when you approach any type of exercise and sports (except for contact sports) slowly and carefully, learning to keep in pace with your body.

The problem in this country is that there is entirely too much misunderstanding about the word *fitness*. It is *not* synonymous with health. You can be physically strong, able to perform difficult motions, and still not be healthy in terms of your cardiovascular or nervous system. The converse is also true: You can be healthy without being able to lift your leg.

This fitness mania produces unnecessary injuries—shin splints, torn ligaments, stress fractures, and insults to the major joints of the limbs and to the spine, to name a few. Even low-impact aerobic dancing, which was designed to replace all the jerky, rapid bouncing and jumping, has produced its own brand of injury. Low-impact aerobics incorporates vigorous arm and shoulder motions, shifting the site of injury from the lower part of the body to the upper. (Potential injuries aside, low-impact is wonderful for older people and a gentler beginning for people who have been inactive; it won't hurt your back, but it also won't do much to improve your shape.)

I'm singling out aerobic dancing because it swept this country like a tornado (leaving injuries in its wake); and became the ultimate craze in a population already crazed by fitness.

I believe exercise should be a way of life, done on a regular basis to maintain health and prevent physical problems. I myself dislike exercising (and despise the word itself), but I am thrilled when I achieve results in such a short time without sustaining any injury. I do not need to be entertained; I just want to feel and look good—to be incredibly fit and in the best possible health—and all of this while being able to stand straight.

Orthopedists are commonly thought of as the first professionals to see if you have back trouble. Like most medical doctors, they tend to take a conventional approach. Some rely on X rays to tell them what's wrong, but many back problems don't show up on X rays. An orthopedist can be valuable in determining if back pain is mechanical or caused by a tumor or an infection. If an orthopedist is a surgeon, there is a greater likelihood that he will consider surgery before exploring other means of treatment.

Family practitioners practice general medicine and would seem to be the logical people to see first if you have back trouble. Depending upon your condition, your family doctor may either choose to treat you himself or refer you to a specialist.

Osteopaths receive a similar education to other medical doctors, but their viewpoint is different. Osteopathy is based on the primary role the musculoskeletal system plays in health. Although osteopaths can prescribe drugs, and in some cases perform surgery, their main method of treatment is a form of manipulation of bones and muscles.

Physiatrists. This is a relatively recent field of specialization, and it may be hard to find a practitioner, particularly if you don't live near a big city. For the back patient, physiatrists seem to combine the best of both worlds: a cross between a physical therapist, movement therapist, and traditional physician. They are trained medical doctors who are more familiar with such natural hands-on methods as exercise, heat, cold, water, sound, and electricity. Rather than prescribing drugs, they prefer to prescribe specific exercises. They never perform surgery. Often they use muscle injections to relax tight or spasmed muscles. In a survey done a few years ago among back pain sufferers, treatment by physiatrists ranked first for both short- and long-term improvement.

Sports medicine doctors. These new specialists have probably increased in direct response to this country's fitness (injury) boom. They treat sports-related injuries, professionals as well as amateur (one doctor can have an entire team as patients!) and believe in exercise, building up muscles with weights, and other physical medicine.

I feel it's a shame that, even in these days of advanced knowledge, some athletes still never concern themselves with their back pains. Somehow, they have been programmed to think that a bad back is the price one pays for this activity. To me, this thinking is totally wrong in light of the fact that we have such excellent ways to prevent injuries and protect the back.

Acupuncturists can be either medical doctors or not. Acupuncture is an ancient Oriental science based on the meridians (energy lines) of the body. Thin needles are inserted on certain points along the meridians to treat specific parts of the body.

My first brush with acupuncture came when I lived in Malaysia.

A neighbor in Penang who was in terrible pain asked me if I would like to go with him and his children to "Took me pain of head gone." I really expected to witness another voodoo ceremony, but as I had been suffering with a migraine headache for two days, I thanked him for his kindness and went along. I was quite taken aback when, instead of being ushered into the ceremony I was bracing myself for, I found myself in a normal office. He lay down on the table, and a man began inserting needles all over his body and twisting them around. I felt sick; I could have used a fainting couch at that point. But, while I thought my friend was suffering, I saw the two men talking and laughing. When we walked out, my friend was very animated, happy and playing with his six-year-old child. In my bewildered state, I had to be assisted to the car.

I didn't have acupuncture in Penang, but I tried it later, when I was in spasm. It helped considerably, but it didn't last. Some people swear that it is the answer for back pain; others have little success. Acupuncturists say that it blocks the pain before it reaches the brain, and in this way does provide at least temporary relief.

Acupuncture is not only used as a treatment for back problems. Because the meridians supposedly influence all the body's functions, an acupuncturist treats a variety of conditions. It has been used to help people stop smoking and as an anesthetic for dental work.

Chiropractors use spinal manipulation as their main tool in treating back pain. Chiropractic is based on the principle that the brain and nervous system transmit the energy that controls all bodily functions. Manipulation of the spine, called adjustments, corrects any subluxation (misalignment of vertebrae). These adjustments can prevent and correct a broad spectrum of ailments and symptoms. Chiropractors don't use drugs or perform surgery. When necessary, they use such aids as electrical muscle stimulation, sound waves, heat therapy, and traction, and usually require X rays before treating patients. Chiropractors are licensed in all fifty states by the same agencies that license medical doctors. Much of their training is concentrated on the spine; they have had great success helping back sufferers and are becoming more popular each year.

My introduction to chiropractic was very dramatic. When I had my first and worst back spasm, I was so incapacitated that, as desperate as I was to lie down, I couldn't get onto the bed. The closest I got was to kneel on the floor and rest my head and torso on the edge. I had been teaching a private student (in my high heels, of course) when the attack occurred. She was extremely frightened and could only think of calling an ambulance. But while we waited (and waited and waited) she was able to reach her chiropractor, who was kind enough to make a house call immediately. He worked on my back for about ten or fifteen minutes, and I managed to get enough relief and release to be able to stand up, with his assistance. Totally bent over, but standing nonetheless. I felt like I had just conquered the world.

There are some people who are still wary of chiropractors, who are afraid they will be hurt. As with all practitioners, it's important to find one you can trust. All my experience with chiropractors has been rewarding and pain-free.

Physical therapists (physiotherapists). Many times, doctors refer their patients to a physical therapist, who has been trained medically. This practitioner treats back problems and related conditions with gentle joint and soft tissue manipulation, heat, cold, exercise, relaxation, massage, range-of-movement therapy, and hydrotherapy. When necessary, physical therapists administer transcutaneous electrical nerve stimulation (TENS), diathermy, and ultrasound. They teach people to correct poor postural habits and teach new movement patterns to help relieve and prevent pain. They play an important role in rehabilitation of the handicapped and disabled.

Occupational therapists. Like physical therapists, occupational therapists are medically trained and take physicians' referrals. They play an important role in rehabilitation of the handicapped and disabled. They help patients learn to live with any limitations caused by physical or mental disabilities, and teach people how to reduce strain and stress while performing the activities of daily living at home, school and work, thereby preventing further complications. Occupational therapists also help choose appropriate self-help and adaptive items and show patients ways to organize and adapt their homes or workplaces to suit their physical needs.

Massage therapists, masseurs, and masseuses. Wherever I went in India, I would see women washing their children, family laundry, and themselves in rivers. I always found it intriguing to see grown women playing in the shallow water, like tiny children in a playground. They laughed, splashed water on one another, and broke into shy, tinkling giggles of embarrassment when they fell into the water. They had such fun chasing each other, while the family laundry floated downstream. (This was far more exciting for me than seeing historical sites.) When they tired of playing, they would sit on the bank, stroking their infants for what seemed like hours. Starting at the feet, they would massage the child's toes, the bottom and top of the feet, the ankle, and all the way up to the scalp. Even the nose was stroked.

The infants loved every second of it. As the mothers stroked and hummed, they cooed and smiled broadly. I felt a little cheated; it was obvious to me that these infants would grow up being very secure, for one of their earliest experiences in the world was that of stroking and love. That's what I feel is one marvelous value of massage, along with the obvious therapeutic ones.

Massage eases muscular pain, releases tight tendons, and relaxes the entire body. The pressure of the massage will depend upon the practitioner and the client. Some people (like me) enjoy really intense massages; others can't handle them. Massage therapists work on specially designed tables, using oil. Massage is not just for people who are wealthy and want to be relaxed. Masseurs are professionals, and must be licensed, like doctors and nurses. *Medical massage* from masseurs who have received medical training can be used on almost all conditions, such as sciatica, scoliosis, lordosis, and bursitis. In fact, seventy-five percent of the patients treated at the well-known Swedish Massage Institute in New York City go there because of back problems. The most common massage techniques are Swedish and shiatsu (Oriental acupressure). Swedish massage, perhaps the best-known technique in this country, involves the use of the entire hand in a variety of strokes over the whole body.

Shiatsu practitioners exert pressure with their thumbs on points in the body corresponding to the meridians used in acupuncture. Sometimes they will even use their feet; no words can adequately describe the sensation of someone walking on your back.

I first came into contact with shiatsu in Japan. It was in a private bathhouse for men, but because I had a special invitation, I was allowed to experience it. A young girl (the only people working in private baths were extremely young girls) approached me. From the outset, I could feel her hostility. She was not programmed to work on females. She began to walk on my back, which felt wonderful, but all of a sudden her dislike burst forth. She started calling me a stupid outsider (in Japanese, of course) and proceeded to jump on my back, like a full-grown male orangutan defending his territory. I felt as though my insides were going to explode. The force was so great, I couldn't even scream for help.

Fortunately, in the West, we don't have this bias. Shiatsu is now available to everyone, is absolutely wonderful (when done with love and care), and should be experienced—but forget it if you're a female in Japan!

Foot reflexology, also called zone therapy, is a system of foot massage based on the principle that all the nerves in the body correspond to specific areas in the feet. The theory is that specific organs, glands, etc., connect to zones in the feet and therefore diseases, ailments, and pain can be treated by placing finger pressure on them.

Touch for Health, Reiki, Jin Shin Jyutsu. For the sake of space, I'm placing these together, although technically they differ quite a bit from one another. What they do have in common is a gentle approach to hands-on treatment of ailments and pain. Using hands therapeutically is ancient, and all of these techniques share some part of that tradition in this way. Practiced by some nurses in hospitals, as well as others, Touch for Health deals with the transfer of energy from the practitioner to the patient, and despite its name does not involve touching at all but rather working on an "energy field" a few inches away from the body. Reiki also deals with energy transfer and works to bring the body into harmony. The Reiki practitioner applies very light pressure with the hands and fingers to certain points where there might be some "blockage." Jin Shin Jyutsu involves releasing tensions that cause various disharmonies (symptoms) in the body. Through gentle touch and understanding of the numerous pulses of the body, Jin Shin works to break up blockages and allow for the flow of healing energy.

Very rarely do these practitioners view what they do as primary care. Instead, they advise patients to see doctors or other specialists and to consider the hands-on treatment as supplementary.

Kinesiology. Practitioners of applied kinesiology test muscles for strength and flexibility through resistance techniques. They use a combination of manipulation, exercise, and massage to relieve pain and improve health. Some chiropractors are trained in applied kinesiology and integrate it into their practice.

Exercise programs. No matter what other helpers you use, I feel a responsible exercise program is essential for sound health in general and for back problems in particular. There are more exercise programs to choose from than you probably will have time even to investigate. The YMCA-YWCA has an excellent program specifically designed for back sufferers. See the introduction to this chapter for more about teachers.

Movement therapists. Movement therapists are concerned with reeducation—replacing inefficient movement patterns with more mechanically sound ones. They teach you how to use your body more efficiently in order to reduce or eliminate pain and any consequent limitation.

Alexander technique and Feldenkrais. These two approaches are placed together because they both deal with retraining the body in postural habits. They have in common reeducating the student in methods of standing, sitting, and lying down so as to avoid or minimize pain. The objective is to encourage self-help.

T'ai chi chuan. This is a gentle, graceful exercise regimen, which originated in China hundreds of years ago. T'ai chi is slow and involves deep concentration and discipline. It can be very effective as a means to reduce stress (one major cause of back pain); it heightens your awareness of the body and fosters relaxation and proper alignment. Probably most important, particularly for older people, is the remarkable way in which it teaches you how to balance the body and calm the mind at the same time.

Every morning at sunrise, down the street from my quarters in Hong Kong (only a narrow canvas hospital stretcher on which I slept), a group of men would practice something beautiful and gentle to the soul. Their ages, I was told, ranged from sixty to eighty. For months I would squat and watch their magnificent, graceful, flowing motions as they went into and came out of positions with perfect balance and harmony. They moved so slowly it seemed as though they were balancing the Empress Dowager's favorite vase on their heads. It looked like a ballet of flamingos walking in shallow water, stalking fish. I never had the courage to ask if I could participate for fear of infringing on their beliefs that women had no place in certain male-oriented rituals. And anyway I looked so puny—like a street urchin—from my worldwide hardships that one of the men could have easily thrashed me with his two-foot-long white beard.

I was extremely fascinated with these elderly men's control of their body and their mastery of balance. It was as though God said, "Float for me in my sky." And because I believed at that time that I was the only Westerner to see this regal posture and gliding flexibility, I felt very blessed.

Years later, in New York, I went with a friend to a "mystery" class. She kept telling me about this "new" technique, which was really ancient, called t'ai chi. I was very confused. I thought this was an American gymnastics class, and I couldn't understand how anything in America—two hundred years old—could be ancient compared to the rest of the world. As I began to participate, a warm rush pulsated through my body, no longer puny. I screamed out loud right in the middle of the class, "How magnificent. Now we Americans can also float in God's sky!"

Yoga. One of the oldest forms of body movement and discipline, this ancient Indian technique employs some of the best stretches you can do. If I had no responsibility in my life, I would be stretching next to some of my friends who spend ninety minutes a day in yoga class. That's one of the difficulties—the time. No doubt in the old days, people took as long as was needed to complete the entire program of yoga positions. It's a shame that everyone doesn't have time now to practice yoga regularly, if even once a week. I think it would be wonderful if classes were streamlined to today's life-style —perhaps cut down to a half hour without sacrificing the basic motions. Many more people could then benefit from this excellent discipline.

Yoga combines motion, meditation, and relaxation and can be extremely valuable for the mind as well as the body. For the back sufferer, yoga should be individualized with a specific program worked out with an instructor. I feel the instructor should have firsthand experience of what it means to suffer from back pain since some yoga positions put incredible pressure on the lower back and neck (the plough and headstands, for example—see pages 144–145), and, in the long run, may contribute to disintegration of discs and severe pain. It's possible that modifications are required for Western life-styles, and in light of current knowledge of the body.

If your priority is to tighten your body or resculpt it, yoga is not an effective exercise. But it is truly valuable for stretching and relaxing the muscles and for quieting the mind.

Back schools. These are fairly recent phenomena, established to meet the needs of the ever-increasing back pain plague. Patients are taught how to control pain through individualized programs, and work either privately or in groups with trained practitioners. Courses are offered by physical therapists and hospitals.

Pain clinics. Pain clinics are not only concerned with the back sufferer; they deal with pain in all areas. They teach the patient techniques of living with the pain, not necessarily how to eliminate it.

10.
Power of the Mind

"Limits of any kind are illusions." —Harry Houdini

There is little dispute these days that the mind and body are totally interconnected; and I am truly thankful for that. Some people seem to be born with a natural talent for controlling their bodies through the mind; others learn it with a great deal of effort; still others don't have a clue about what it means.

Whether scientifically provable or not, the mind can have such power over the body as to alleviate pain and help heal physical conditions. The converse is unfortunately even more common—the mind can also create pain and disease. Back problems are no exception. In fact, there are some very reputable practitioners (including medical doctors) who strongly believe most back pain (as well as other pain in the body) is induced by the mind and can therefore be eliminated by it. In my own teaching experience, I had students who came in with skeletal and other body problems that I discovered were subconsciously brought on by them. I came to this understanding because the problems would clear up when I dealt with them in an encouraging, caring, positive manner.

Relaxation and visualization are ways to tap into the subconscious. Meditation is one way to practice relaxing. It's also an excellent stress-reducer; it allows you to quiet the mind, which in turn can soothe and heal the body. It is a known fact that meditation can control such autonomic nervous system functions as blood pressure. There may be real value in employing meditative techniques for stress-related back problems. This doesn't require elaborate or mystical measures; it can be accomplished by closing your office or kitchen door, sitting erect, closing your eyes, consciously relaxing every part of your body, and shutting out all interference. In this state, you can visualize anything you want; for instance, if you want your back healed, see and feel that it's being healed.

I found a book (*Feeling Is the Secret* by Neville) many years ago that has helped me and others enormously with a practical means of visualizing total wellness. What you think or visualize in the period right before falling asleep is very important. The author puts forth the theory that the subconscious mind, during sleep, picks up these thoughts and materializes these impressions in your waking state. He writes: "Night after night, you should assume the feeling of being, having, and witnessing that which you wish to be, possess and see manifested. Never go to sleep feeling discouraged or dissatisfied. Never sleep in the consciousness of failure."

Here are examples of both positive and negative thought. If you think right before you drift off, "My life is ruined. I'm broke. I won't be able to support my family," when you wake in the morning, you will find yourself still thinking the same way. You're exhausted before you begin the day. This has a chain reaction effect: Because you're so debilitated, you become even more negative, and do things as though you were suffering from sleep deprivation. Thoughts, negative or positive, have this way of exacerbating a situation. Suppose you get a slight pain, then become anxious about it. Before long the pain has become more intense. You get more anxious, and the cycle can be never-ending, until you break it yourself, through your awareness of the relationship between the conscious mind, the subconscious mind, and the body.

The good news is that you can do the same thing with positive emotions. If you listen to beautiful music, or the sounds of the ocean or trees gently blowing in the wind, or even inspirational programs (all of which are available on tape), and you visualize yourself happy, free of any physical problems you may have, then you will probably wake up the morning with a sense of well-being, your body feeling lighter and your spirits more buoyant.

Such is the power of the subconscious. A doctor told me about a man who was having an operation for a particular problem. While the patient was under anesthesia, the attending physicians were discussing the case of another patient with an entirely different problem. The man recovered from surgery, but two months later he developed the *exact* problem, to the *exact* degree, as the patient whose case had been discussed during his operation. This is one dramatic example of the power of suggestion, but I'm sure all of you have heard similar stories. A friend of mine heard so many of them that she decided, whether it was scientific or not, she was going to accept them as true. In the hospital for a minor surgical procedure, she wrote the following note and pinned it on the front of her gown prior to being wheeled into the operating room: "To my team: Would you kindly speak out loud to me and my subconscious mind while you're operating on us. We would appreciate hearing how well things are going and that now we are in perfectly good health, thanks to your expertise and efficiency. Love, Lynn. P.S.: See you when I wake up." She later told me the surgical team really appreciated her including them; and she is firmly convinced that her awareness of the role of her subconscious contributed to her excellent recovery.

It is not only during the state of sleep or unconsciousness that the mind has such an impact on the body. We send messages to the body throughout our waking hours, often without being aware of it. Our body language is more communicative than our words. You can tell a lot about how a person feels or what he or she is thinking by the posture, hunch of the shoulders, or way of walking. For instance, to get to my exercise area, one has to walk down a long corridor. From over a decade of listening to feet, I have become quite adept at ascertaining what emotional state my students' walks represented, before I even saw them.

The power the mind has to fulfill an expectation is something I have witnessed all over the world, from voodoo to walking barefoot on hot coals to mind control. The mind's power is accepted by so many cultures that I'm bewildered when I'm told that it's mystical nonsense. While traveling in the Central African bush on horseback, I accompanied a friend who worked for the government. One of his jobs was administering supplies to the different tribes. He was close to the chiefs, and well trusted and respected. When we reached a village, there would be a line of people waiting to tell him about their ailments (ranging from bilharzia to stubbed toes) so that he could give them medication. I couldn't help noticing that all the pills looked alike—the same shape, the same color. The strangest thing was that everyone got better very quickly, regardless of what was wrong with them. At the time I had never heard the term *placebo effect*, but I was a firsthand witness to it. These people firmly believed that the medication would work—and it did for that very reason, despite the fact that it was the exact same pill for a variety of ailments.

Emotions can easily trigger physical responses, even when you pride yourself on being in control. Here's an embarrassing real-life story: I would always go into spasm, for no apparent reason, two days before I flew home to Savannah. (I could not figure it out because I had given up my high heels.) The only way I could sit on the plane was to be laced into a back brace, and the spasm persisted throughout my stay, no matter how long I was there. There was a particular woman back home with whom I despised speaking; but because of the pain, I was incapable of socializing with her. In this way I received a negative reward from my pain. Twenty minutes into the flight back to New York, I would be conscious of feeling the pain starting to ease. After three such trips, I began to analyze the situation and realized that I created these spasms because I was too much of a coward; too afraid of hurting her feelings, to tell her I didn't wish to speak with her.

Another time I had a date with someone. About five minutes before he was to arrive, I realized that under no circumstances did I want to share my time with him. But I could not bring myself to be honest with him; I was feeling too guilty about the inconvenience I was causing him. So instead I went into spasm. In that way, I avoided a confrontation and the possibility of being thought of as rude and inconsiderate. My subconscious fully cooperated with my conscious;

in transferring my thoughts to my body, it gave me a legitimate excuse for not being brave. Similar situations have occurred many times in my life, so that now when I feel some bodily discomfort for no apparent reason, I begin to question why. And if it has to do with fear of communication, I take the risk. It's worth not suffering physically.

If you suppress emotions and don't express them, they will have to be released in another way, and that way is usually through your body. You create this scenario and your body acts it out.

Stress affects the immune system, which prevents the body from fighting disease. Stressful emotions will invariably attack a person's weakest, most vulnerable areas; my years of teaching have made me a firm believer in this. In my case (and many others), it is the lower back; with other people it's the stomach, neck, head, etc. It goes even further: You can have specific areas of pain within a general area— for instance, your upper back may be affected by money worries, your lower back by personal relationships, and on and on. Test this out yourself. The next time you feel pain somewhere, ask yourself honestly, What was I thinking or feeling or doing just before the onset? Try to remember the last time you felt the same pain or discomfort. Was there any connection with this time? By bringing this awareness into your conscious mind, you could be on the way to preventing recurrences, and you might discover that you can alter your attitude in general so that your body is not always at the mercy of your subconscious.

There are practical ways to express your emotions and use stress constructively. Negative stress should be handled before it becomes destructive. Take crying. Crying is one of the most spiritual gifts you can give yourself. One reason I love being a female is that it's more acceptable to cry. Men have been conditioned by society to believe that crying, even in private, is not manly. (I'm pleased to see this changing.) It is truly liberating to cry or express anger or fear. When we carry these feelings around, it's like Atlas carrying the world on his shoulders. I keep thinking of the character Liza Minelli played in *Cabaret*. She knew the train schedule and would station herself on the underpass while the train was going over the bridge. At the precise moment the noise of the train would drown her out, she would scream from her toes. When I saw the movie, I was quite surprised; I thought I was the only person who did such things. You may feel like a fool at first, but try using your pillow as a whipping post—scream into it or fiercely pound it. Releasing tensions and negative emotions in this way will make you feel like all your sins have been cleansed from your body and soul. And remember to scream from your feet!

Stress can be a powerful positive force if you know how to use it. Take it as an opportunity to empower yourself. It often plays a primary role in motivation. For instance, many people have trouble completing tasks unless they have a deadline. The difference between constructive stress and negative stress is that the latter causes *dis*tress, which can lead to *dis*orders.

Stress can be caused by many factors, not the least of which is boredom, which in turn leads to fatigue and irritability. Exercise has a way of transforming all stress (regardless of the cause) into usable energy, making you look, think, and feel better. You feel like you're in control of your body, and that actually helps to relieve the stress. The exercise does not have to be rapid or strenuous. Do what feels good—just get moving! You can walk briskly or do the slow, deep-muscle exercises outlined in this book.

By understanding and training the incredible power of your mind, you can begin to participate in your own healing.

11.

You're Never Too Young or Too Old

CHILDREN

All the emphasis on fitness today seems to be for adults, not children. These days, most parents are in better shape than their children.

I think this is a crime. Parents and teachers are in the best position to help forge important lifelong habits.

For parents, this opportunity comes even before a baby starts walking. First of all, there are the shoes. What possible reason would you have for putting those hard, uncomfortable structures on developing, delicate little feet—especially when they're not even walking? Unless a child has specific medical problems (such as I did), there is no point in restricting those early motions. If you must cover their feet, make sure the shoes are soft and flexible enough to encourage movement of the toes, ankles, etc. There is no sense in pushing the body to do things before its organic time. I have a real dislike for baby walkers, those plastic prisons that tend to make children walk on their toes before they can walk naturally. The continual use of walkers might deprive the baby of his or her natural inclination to crawl. Crawling is an important stage for infants, because it develops strength, particularly in the shoulders, as well as spatial skills. Another problem is overeager parents who hold their infants' arms to force them to walk before they are naturally ready; jerking up a child by the arms or swinging the child can be potentially dangerous because the shoulder joint isn't that stable and the arm muscles are not developed enough to protect that area.

Before leaving the subject of infants, I'd like to speak about massage. In the chapter called People Helpers, I told a story about watching Indian mothers massage their babies. It seems that the sense of touch is the first one that develops in the womb—before sight and hearing—and is the predominant sensation at birth. It's no wonder that massaging a baby can have such positive therapeutic effects as stimulating the respiratory, circulatory, and gastrointestinal functions, as well as playing a critical role in the bonding between child and parent—something that could influence the rest of the child's life.

Parents can be excellent role models. Take posture—standing, walking, and sitting. It is very easy to teach correct posture to a very young child. Make it a game; correct each other's posture, whenever necessary. This will reinforce the child's awareness (as well as your own). After a while, good posture will become natural and automatic. If you wait until your child is older, it will probably be a task you will give up on; it's just too draining for you and the child. If you start before they begin school, you may stand a chance of making an impression. It's never too early to show a child how to sit up straight instead of slumping; how to bring the food to one's mouth instead of bending the head and shoulders over to reach the plate; how to stand erect without sticking out the abdomen or buttocks; how to lift objects by bending the knees. All these positions will start a child on the right road to protecting his or her back. After all, back problems can start at any age.

Paying attention to posture teaches your child to be conscious of the body, but the effects are more far-reaching than that. Posture is an immediate indication of how you feel about yourself and how you relate to others. Your table manners and carriage are passports to the world for the rest of your life; the way you hold yourself can make the difference between getting a desired job or not.

School can play a major part in a child's physical development and fitness from the very beginning. It's very difficult for a child to sit in one position for long periods of time. There should be activity breaks every hour. Some easy t'ai chi chuan motion (for balance), simple stretches, or gentle jumping jacks right next to the desk can be fun and will certainly help to rejuvenate them and make them more alert. Something so simple can be very powerful. Walking around the room with a book on the head will not take much time and can help posture tremendously. Activities can vary each hour; the important thing is to keep them moving. And as early as the first grade, children should learn about their organs and their skeletal structure. Preschools and nurseries do a much better job than the elementary schools and upper grades; because play is such an intrinsic part of the early school years, there's a great deal of motion—jumping, skipping, running—as well as using the body to act out stories, songs, and rhymes. The amount of exercise seems to decrease with the age of the child.

The greatest challenge comes when children have "gym." It's almost a trauma for some, mostly because it's so boring and so far removed from the real world of fitness and health. There's a lot of hanging around and learning rules of games they'll probably never play; or else they're pushed to compete so they can become great athletes (which most of them will never be). Physical education can be made exciting with a little imagination on the part of the school, but too often the school sees it as an unnecessary interruption to learning, which does nothing to improve the mind. Studies have shown that when children were given time for this activity every day, even though their classroom time was reduced, they performed better academically than those children who had physical education only two or three times a week.

Children with hypermobile joints (misnamed "double-jointed") used to be chosen for ballet and certain sports. Now the trend is just the opposite: Schools should be testing children for hypermobility and discouraging those who have it (particularly in the knees) from participating in activities that have a high risk of injury.

One of the big culprits is television. Time that might be better spent exercising or participating in sports is spent in front of the set, just sitting and wasting away. The result is inactivity, dullness of mind, and the potential for obesity. Childhood obesity is a serious matter. Studies show that one quarter of American children are obese; and about 75 percent of obese ten- to thirteen-year-olds will be obese adults. Sadly, it's not unusual to see nine-year-old children already on reducing diets. Interestingly, only 41 percent of seven-year-olds have the same potential for obesity, which seems to imply that the earlier you limit children's TV time (and increase their physical activity), the better their chances of not developing "fat habits" that could lead to complications (including bad backs) in adulthood. In fact, summer camps designed to thin children down are a big business. The problem is that some camps tend to push the children past their limitations. Emotionally and physically they are pressured to lose weight within a specified period of time and are made to do routines that place undue pressure on the lower back.

The problem of childhood and adolescent un-fitness has serious implications for future generations. It's time that parents, teachers, and school administrators remember that at any age the ancient philosophy is still true: The body and mind are one.

OLDER PEOPLE

No matter what your age, it's a wonderful, powerful feeling to know that you look and feel good. You feel that you're a part of life and not just dragging yourself through each day.

I was being considered for a big national promotion aimed for people in my age group. The woman in charge said, "They're going to love your energy—especially since you're hitting fifty." A few weeks later I received a surprising phone call: They decided not to use me because I didn't think or act old, and they were afraid the audience wouldn't be able to relate to me as a peer. I'm still not sure I know what that means; but I chose to interpret it as the most wonderful compliment. (Am I supposed to now think of myself as a teenager?!)

Just exactly what is "old"? What are the qualifications for being a member of the old-age club? If it's any fun, I definitely want to be a member. And what is young? Young to me is something I never want to experience again in my life. I didn't want to be a member of that club when it was my birthright. Our attachment to the numbers gives them an unwarranted power. For instance, I once overheard a man say about a woman he knew, "She's aging—she's forty-five." I knew for a fact that this man was a good fifteen years younger than the woman he was speaking about, but he looked worn out and older than she. I wanted to clobber him. The way we allow the numbers to lie to us!

I feel that the older one gets, the more essential it is to work the body. Aside from the obvious advantages for combating osteoporosis, exercise may reduce the risk of obesity, high blood pressure, and heart disease. It also helps you to have a positive outlook toward life. Motion is healing. With age, the fluid around the spinal discs tends to diminish. Exercise keeps it moving. The drying-out process is not limited to the spine; joints and ligaments have less flexibility (compare a tree branch in spring to one in the winter). Stiffness is not only a result of aging; it can happen from lack of activity.

Instead of seeing this natural change as depressing, it can be taken as a challenge. One doesn't have to join the ranks of the marathoners to become physically active. You can start with whatever you're capable of doing and move on. Not getting stuck in your age means being able to accept certain limitations without letting them defeat you. You may think you have to limit your exercise to gardening or golf (with a cart, of course). But it isn't true; you can do something more physical, like stretching or tap dancing. For instance, my mother's doctor told her that if she had not been exercising in her later years, she would already be in a wheelchair, bedridden, or worse. Now, at almost eighty, she is acting out a lifelong fantasy: to tap-dance. Doing "real" exercise will enable you to do everything else (including golf) with more ease and skill.

You must be sensible about exercise when you're older. Strenuous exercise may be more damaging for older people than younger ones. Do not attempt the exercises you did when you were under thirty-five, or those you see younger people doing, without professional direction. In approaching an exercise program, a good way to test your ability is to walk through the motions, rather than doing them at the usual pace. Remember that you are more prone to dizziness and losing your balance. Avoid exercises that require you to take your head back, close your eyes while in motion, and jump around too hard and fast. Ease into a program, and do it consistently. If you exercise erratically, you will not progress well but will keep having to start over. Above all, do not be discouraged.

Be sure to choose something that is enjoyable; exercise is not a bitter pill to be swallowed quickly. Instead, it provides wonderful opportunities to socialize with people of all ages, which helps to keep you young, and to play. We've been conditioned to believe that being

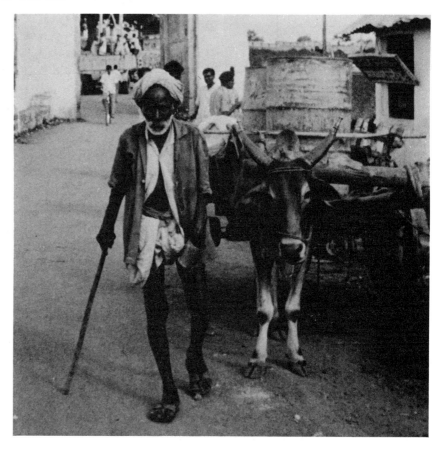

In almost all the countries I visited, it seemed that the women of a certain age were all bent over while the men of the same age stood more erect. I always took it for granted that women's bodies become more bent with age. Maybe it has something to do with the fact that donkeys and women are the main means of transportation for heavy loads; or maybe it's the higher incidence of osteoporosis. Notice the lovely posture of this man, who was almost ninety.

an adult means taking on enormous responsibilities and that adults don't play. Everyone needs play throughout their lives. The wondrous part of growing old is to stop bearing the weight of these responsibilities and to use your leisure time to participate in life instead of waiting for it to end.

I'm so tired of people telling me, on the subject of exercise, "I'm too old," or "It's too late for me." As long as you can move, it's not too late. Every year, there are more inspiring stories of men and women in their eighties and even nineties finishing long-distance races, or working out in gyms or at home, or riding their bikes as their only means of transportation; one group of women, all over sixty, are cheerleaders (complete with traditional outfits) for a high school team. Age allows you to do the most outlandish things. You'll probably be classified as an eccentric—take advantage of it. Do whatever you want; you deserve it. You've led a life of accomplishment of which you and others can be proud. And you came through it. Now is the time to give yourself a wonderful gift—the total aliveness that comes from moving.

12.

A Brief
Anatomy Lesson

The purpose of this chapter is to provide you with a simplified understanding of the anatomy of the back, and to familiarize you with some of the terms used throughout this book.

BONES

Bones are the supportive framework (along with the muscles) of the body that make movement possible. There are 206 of them in the body. They are all rigid and unbending.

The *skeleton* is a jointed framework of bones and cartilages for supporting body weight. It provides the muscles with levers to move the body (movement); supports the surrounding tissues (weight-bearing); protects organs within the skull, thoracic (rib) cage, and pelvis (protection).

The *spinal column* is a curved column of bones that gives stability to the torso; allows movement in all directions; supports the skull, shoulder girdle, and rib cage; transmits body weight to the pelvis; acts as a shock absorber to cushion jolts and jars; provides attachment for numerous muscles and ligaments; protects the spinal cord. It consists of 25 separate vertebrae, cylindrical-shaped bones that are stacked on top of one another. Each vertebra is joined by five separate articulations connected by ligaments and muscles. Several bony processes (projections) stick out from the back of the spine. These projections articulate with others on adjacent vertebrae and form the areas where back muscles attach, allowing the spine to bend and twist. The spine moves in four ways:

1. Flexion (forward bending)
2. Extension or hyperextension (backward bending)
3. Lateral flexion (sideward bending)
4. Rotation (twisting)

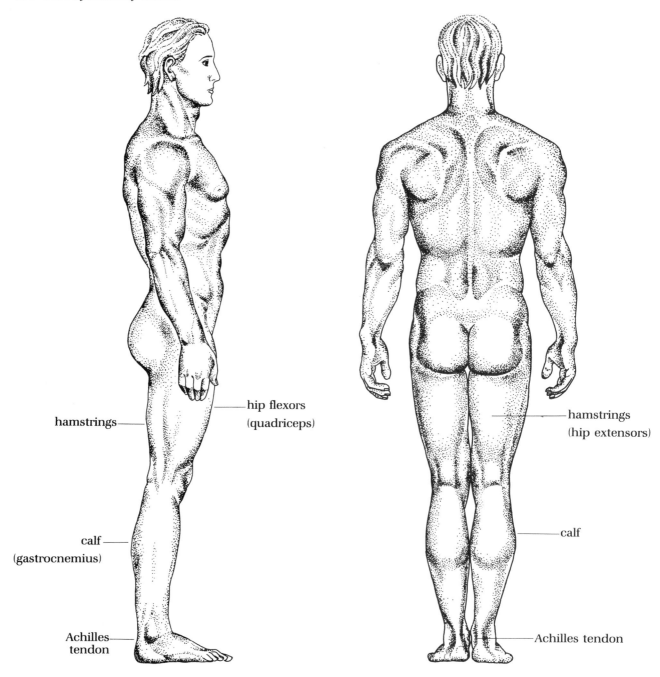

hamstrings

hip flexors
(quadriceps)

hamstrings
(hip extensors)

calf
(gastrocnemius)

calf

Achilles
tendon

Achilles tendon

Looking from the side, the spine has four natural curves in each of the following areas:

Cervical: There are seven cervical vertebrae, which support the skull and neck. The first two (named C1 and C2; also called the atlas and axis) support and rotate the head and allow the most range of motion.

Thoracic: There are twelve thoracic vertebrae (named T1–12) which articulate with twelve pairs of ribs. These support the thorax (which holds the heart, lungs, and other organs). The thoracic vertebrae are largely immobile; their main function is protection of the vital organs.

Lumbar: There are five lumbar (lower back) vertebrae (named L1–5), which carry a great portion of the body weight. The large

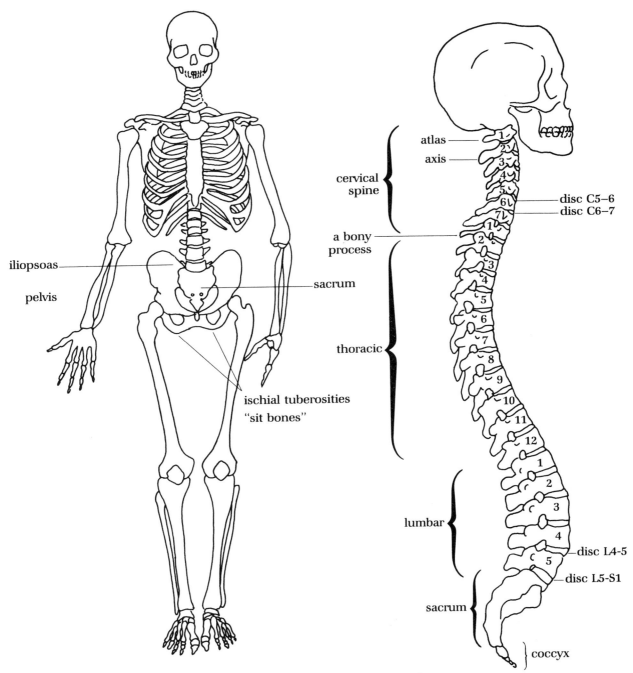

atlas

axis

cervical
spine

disc C5–6
disc C6–7

a bony
process

thoracic

lumbar

disc L4-5

disc L5-S1

sacrum

coccyx

iliopsoas

pelvis

sacrum

ischial tuberosities
"sit bones"

muscles (iliopsoas) attach here. L3, 4, and 5 are most vulnerable to injury and are usually associated with lower back pain.

Sacral: The sacrum is the connecting structure between the spine and the hips and legs. There are five sacral vertebrae, which are fused (connected together so that they do not move independently). These transmit the weight of the body to the hips and together form the pelvic girdle.

Coccyx: There are two to four vertebrae at the base of the spinal column. These are also fused; together with the sacrum, they are the remnant of the vestigial "tail" of our forebears. Most of the pelvic ligament connects to the coccyx.

JOINTS

Joints are at the juncture where two or more bones meet. There are several types of joints in the body. Among the most common types are gliding, hinge, and ball-and-socket. Joints determine both the range and freedom of motion of a limb or other body part.

The ends of bones are covered with a smooth, shiny material called *cartilage*. This is spongy, gelatinous, and mostly water. Cartilage cushions the joints and protects them from excessive pressure, jolts, and jars. It allows them to move easily. Joints are enclosed in a capsule, the lining of which produces a fluid for lubrication, which helps to reduce friction and wear and tear.

The range of motion of various joints can go from very wide to quite narrow, depending upon the type of joint and how loose the ligaments are. Other factors that influence the range of motion are strength and flexibility of the muscles. Weight-bearing and pressure keep joints healthy by forcing fluid through them—hence the importance of activity using the weight of the body. If you move beyond the joints' "normal" range of motion, the ligaments can overstretch or tear. Age and heredity can also determine joint range.

The knee joint is the most complex in the body and a major engineering feat: It has to flex, slide, and rotate; how many hinges can do that? The knee is comprised of two long bones and a kneecap, held together by seven ligaments (some crisscrossing each other). These are surrounded and protected by three groups of muscles: the quadriceps (front thigh), hamstrings (back thigh), and gastrocnemius (calf). The knee joint is made up of very thick cartilage and cushioning sacs, which are needed for protection and efficiency of movement. The kneecaps protect the knee joint and increase the power of the quadriceps (front thigh) to straighten the knee.

The knee is most frequently injured in sports and other strenuous activities such as some forms of dancing. It is constantly subjected to stress and abuse because so much mobility is required of it. It also provides great stability for the entire body.

Women are prone to more knee injuries because of their wider hips, which require the quadriceps to attach to the kneecaps at a sharper angle.

Everyone should take great care not to misuse or overuse the knee. Particularly taxing are the repetitive deep-knee bends that are often part of weight-lifting programs and other exercise regimens. Avoid locking the knees.

My stretches are wonderful exercises for knees and legs. However, if you feel any pain, check with a doctor before continuing them.

DISCS

Discs lie between the vertebrae. They act as cushions to eliminate any friction, as well as adding mobility to the spine. They are equal to about one third the entire length of the spine. Inside the center of each disc space is a gelatinlike substance, mostly liquid, which allows it to act as a shock absorber and gives the spine its flexibility. The center of each disc is surrounded by layers of elastic bands, or fibers, that crisscross each other.

If the fluid in a disc dries up, problems occur, such as stiffness and possibly vertebral fusion. Movement encourages the flow of fluid in the discs, which is one of the reasons that it's so important to keep active. Discs are named for the vertebrae they lie between. L4-5, L5-S1 are the discs in the lower spine most likely to herniate. In the neck C5-6 and C6-7 have similar vulnerability.

NERVES

Nerves are rooted in the spinal cord and pass through an opening between and behind the vertebrae. A diseased or misaligned disc, bone, or other tissue in the spine can affect nerve roots by causing pressure on them (commonly referred to as a pinched nerve) or pulling it into a stretched position, leading to pain. The sciatic nerve is the longest nerve in the body (see page 175 for problems associated with it).

LIGAMENTS

Ligaments are thick, dense, and tough fibers that attach bone to bone and hold joints together. They are flexible but not very elastic; and they have little involvement in moving the limbs. When ligaments tear, they must be repaired by surgery. If not repaired, joint instability will result, which may lead to further damage to the joint. Another cause of joint instability is overstretching of a ligament. Because a ligament is not elastic, it may loosen and will not return to its normal length. If it is overstretched, it will not return to its original length. A network of many ligaments holds the vertebrae, sacrum, and pelvis together.

TENDONS

Tendons are the dense and tough ends of muscles that attach the muscle to the bone. They are more elastic than ligaments but can still tear. You must exercise regularly to keep them healthy, as there is very little direct blood supply to them.

As we know, movement in general is very important in slowing down the aging process. Contraction and relaxation of muscles, tendons, and ligaments, and working the joints forces the nutrients to move through the tissues, keeping them healthy and supple, thereby diminishing the effects of age or inactivity.

MUSCLES

There are over four hundred voluntary muscles in the body. Muscles are made up of contractile fibers, which are elastic in that they can lengthen and shorten. Nerves originate in the brain and travel down the spinal cord and out to each muscle. In general, muscles don't function individually, but rather as groups (called antagonists and agonists). All muscles are attached to the spine, either directly or indirectly. Even those not located in the back can greatly influence back pain. The following groups of muscles work together as a team and are all needed for sound back health and support of the spine.

1. Abdominal muscles support the abdominal organs. Additionally, even though they are in the front of the body, they provide support for the back.
2. Spinal extensor muscles are many layers of varying sizes, which provide support in the back and keep the torso erect.
3. Side, or lateral, muscles provide support on the side and control side to side movement.
4. Hip muscles affect movement of the pelvis and therefore influence the spine. The hip extensors, in particular, determine the lumbar (lordotic) curve and, with the hip flexors, greatly affect your ability to maintain good posture.

13.

Some Common Causes of Back Pain

In this chapter I've briefly outlined some of the most frequent causes of back pain other than infections, fractures, and tumors. Stress and other psychological factors are discussed on pages 159–162.

SCIATICA

Sciatica is an irritation of the sciatic nerve. The two sciatic nerves, one down the back of each leg, are the longest nerves in the body, and their roots originate from the lower lumbar vertebra. If this nerve is pinched or irritated from a variety of causes—herniated disc (primary), exercise, lifting, or stress—you'll probably feel the pain radiate down the back of one or both legs. Sciatica can also be brought on by tumors, infections, injuries, bony spurs, degenerative conditions such as arthritis, and even muscle spasms. Beware of the shift pedal in your car; the constant pumping motion of the leg will sorely aggravate an existing sciatic condition. Other things that make it worse are straight leg raises, straight knee toe touches, bending improperly, sitting too long at a stretch, crossing your legs—in fact, anything that might cut off the circulation to that area. Even coughing or sneezing can bring on a sciatica attack.

Treatments for acute sciatica depend on the specific cause and can include ice; a combination of ice and heat; rest; loosening and strengthening muscles; and even medication. The condition can be prevented by stretching and strengthening muscles affecting the lower back to increase flexibility of the spine, good postural habits, reduction of stress, and weight control.

DISC PROBLEMS

Disc problems are at the top of the list of causes of back pain. There are numerous problems associated with spinal discs. These are among the most common caused by deterioration of the discs:

Slipped disc is the popular name for a condition that is really herniated or prolapsed disc. Discs are held firmly in place by two vertebrae, so in actuality they cannot slip. There is a high internal pressure within the core of the disc, which is the reason it can act as a shock absorber. Think of it as a water-filled inner tube inside a tire. When the fibers surrounding the center of the disc deteriorate, the material in the center expands through the weakened area, causing a bulge, which in turn may press on a nerve, resulting in discomfort and other symptoms. Depending on its location, the symptoms may involve cramping, spasm, numbness and tingling, muscle weakness, even bowel and bladder problems. They may come on suddenly, but the cause probably has been building up for a period of time. A strenuous move such as lifting something heavy (while bending and twisting), a sports activity, or even something as simple as a sneeze can cause an acute onset.

It's not surprising that disc problems are age-related. Up to the age of twenty-five, injury from sports is the most common cause of back trouble, and any damage to discs is related to those injuries. As people grow older, wear, tear, and stress become the main factors, and the discs are good indicators of this sorry situation.

The discs that are most likely to herniate are the last two of the lumbar spine (L4-5, L5-S 1—see pages 170–171) and the last two of the cervical spine (C5-6 and C6-7—see page 170). In the case of the lumbar spine, the vulnerability is caused by its proximity to the sacrum, which is a series of fused vertebrae that don't move and have no cushioning. Because the sacrum cannot help to absorb shocks and jolts, all the stress is passed on to the lumbar area. This is aggravated because we carry most of our weight in the lower lumbar area; we also, incorrectly, bend from there instead of from the hips.

The treatment most often prescribed is rest, strengthening exercises (particularly the abdominals for the lumbar region), physical therapy, lumbar limbering exercises such as the pelvic wave, and support apparatus. Be certain to get a proper diagnosis, however, as exercising may in some cases aggravate a herniated disc, causing the pain and, in the extreme, surgery may be necessary. Surgery is usually performed where there is intractable pain, progressive neurological signs, and bowel or bladder impairment; pain alone is not considered sufficient cause. Most disc surgery involves removal of the disc via a small opening in the bone. This procedure is known as a laminectomy. Fusion is rare these days. The good news is that 95 percent of disc problems can be resolved without surgery.

ABNORMAL CURVATURES OF THE SPINE: SCOLIOSIS, LORDOSIS, KYPHOSIS

In the 1940's hardly anything was mentioned about scoliosis. I now know that I had scoliosis during that period, but never even heard the term until I was a grown woman.

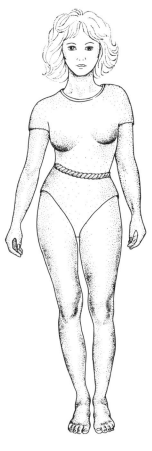

My right hip was higher than my left even as a child—so much so that the hems on all of my dresses and pants (including school uniforms) had to be taken up more on the left side in order to be straight. Before I learned the advantages of sitting down at a party (see page 49), I would always stand with my left leg bent to ensure that my hips looked even.

It became worse as I grew older, but I wasn't aware that one of the reasons I always suffered lower back pain might be the situation with my hips. I assumed it was natural, especially because my mother and father have the same imbalance. Then, one evening as I was preparing to go to a formal affair, a friend of mine said, "Callan, you can't wear that tight dress. It looks dreadful on you—your body is too crooked." When I looked in the mirror, I gasped. I looked as though I had been carrying babies on my right hip for forty years nonstop and they had a permanent resting place there. To put it mildly, I was an hysterical maniac. Instead of going to the party (I could never allow anyone to see me that lopsided!) the next day I went to the specialist who could give me the earliest appointment. His response was the first of a long line of negative prognoses: "Nothing could correct the curvature or make your hips even at your age. You're just too old."

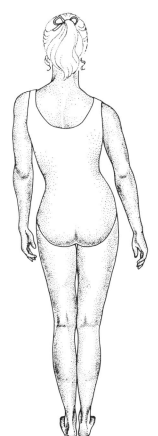

My feminine vanity wouldn't allow me to accept this. Somehow I would find a way (or a person) to correct this condition, but for the time being I forgot about it—until it became apparent to me that many of my new students had very stiff backs. To help them, I started doing a stretch I had developed (along with the rest of my Callanetics exercises) that was based on a particular kind of spinal manipulation (see page 153). It made the entire spine feel wonderful and more flexible. What I didn't realize at the time was that it could help to make the hips even. When I began to do it regularly with my students (and with my heart and soul), I noticed after a few months that for the first time in my life I had even hips. It was as though I had received a beautiful gift of new beginnings from life. (And the tailor no longer makes money from me!)

According to a recent study, scoliosis affects about 10 percent of the population, worldwide, but most cases are so slight that treatment is usually not required.

There are major differences of opinion when it comes to both the cause and treatment of scoliosis. Some practitioners take the position that nothing can be done for the curvature and only a minimal amount for the pain; others feel that both can be improved by a combination of treatment and exercise. Some say just exercise; others say just eliminate the stress. What works for one person may not be the answer for another. Just because I and a lot of other people were helped by my exercises doesn't necessarily mean you'll derive the same benefits. However, even someone with the worst case of scoliosis should do some form of gentle stretching. Use the following discussion to help make your choices regarding treatment. As for me, I'm willing to let everyone argue it out as I go on my merry way, swinging my even hips in my "old age."

Scoliosis derives from the Greek word meaning "crooked." As you know from the previous discussion of anatomy, the spine has four natural curves. The curvature in scoliosis is abnormal in that it is sideward, or S-shaped. Scoliosis occurs most often in the upper back (thoracic) area.

There are three types of scoliosis: functional, structural, or congenital.

Functional scoliosis is usually caused by a mechanical problem such as a shorter leg, back muscle tightness, or spasm and usually can be eliminated with treatment—a lift in the shoe, for example, to make the legs more even, or one that relieves spasms.

Structural scoliosis may be caused by injury, infection, a neurological condition, a disease such as poliomyelitis, muscle imbalance, or for an unknown (idiopathic) reason, which accounts for the largest number of cases (80 to 90 percent). Structural scoliosis mostly affects girls during their early teen years. It appears the cause may be hereditary; it is not due to bad posture or other poor habits.

Congenital scoliosis is due to a malformation of the vertebrae before birth. This is very rare (only about 2 percent of cases).

Several forms of treatment for scoliosis are currently available. Although there is, supposedly, no cure for structural scoliosis, there are ways to keep it from worsening and to relieve the pain which may occur later as a result of it.

Exercise may not correct scoliosis, but in most cases it can help to minimize the pain and help you to function better. Many of the exercises outlined in this book are the same ones recommended for scoliosis, particularly the pelvic wave, which strengthens the abdominal muscles, and hanging from a countertop or bar, which stretches the spine and helps relieve muscle tightness.

Some back exercises may be too strenuous for scoliosis. But if you use your intuition, you will know what your body is dictating and will probably learn not to overstretch. None of the exercises in this book will be harmful if you have scoliosis; some are even specifically designed for it. *However, extreme care must be taken to go very slowly and gently, without forcing; and to stop at the point of discomfort.* Younger scoliosis sufferers can do the exercises in any order, but older people should start with the chapter Stretches for Bad Backs first.

After *Callanetics* was published, I received letters from people with scoliosis who informed me that my exercises were the only ones they could do without experiencing pain or discomfort.

Bracing is most commonly used to prevent the curvature from

getting worse, although it doesn't correct what is already there. The one usually prescribed is the Milwaukee brace, which must be worn twenty-three hours a day for years. It is especially effective for growing children.

Electrical muscle stimulation is claimed to be effective for a moderate curve. The problem is that doctors may wait too long before prescribing it. Electrodes are placed over the area needing stimulation and left on all night. The use of this treatment reportedly makes a brace unnecessary. Electrical muscle stimulation has been around for a while, but more recently it is being used on a wider scale. However, long-term results are not available as there have been no studies undertaken. Some practitioners question its effectiveness.

Surgery is, of course, the most extreme treatment and should only be considered as a last resort (when bracing is ineffective and the curve continues to progress), and even then only after receiving at least two affirmative opinions. It may involve spinal fusion with steel rods. Surgery to correct a severe case of scoliosis is a delicate undertaking and, when successful, extremely helpful.

Parents should check their children often during the growing years for signs of scoliosis; the earlier it is recognized, the more effective the treatment will be. The problem with diagnosing the syndrome in children is that they rarely complain of pain—especially because initially they have none in the upper back. Testing is usually done through a school screening program (mandatory in most states). You should also ask your pediatrician to check your child for signs.

There are several ways you can check for scoliosis at home:

- See if the spine is crooked.
- Have the child bend forward and look for a slight hump or irregularity in the rib cage.
- While the child is standing, look for any difference in symmetry in both sides of the body, such as one shoulder or hip higher than the other; or one breast higher than the other.
- Look for differences in adjusting waistline, hemline, or pants leg.
- Check to see if there is any indication of round shoulders. This condition, known as kyphosis, is another form of curvature, in this case an abnormal forward curve of the upper back.
- Also check for swayback, which is an abnormal lordosis—too much curve in hyperextension of the lower back. Lordosis occurs when the vertebrae in the lower back directly above the pelvis are pulled too far forward. It can also be caused by overdevelopment of the psoas muscle (common to ballet dancers). Lordosis can usually be corrected by increasing the flexibility of the lower back and pelvic area, particularly with pelvic wave motions.

If any of these tests prove positive, consult a back specialist. The earlier you begin treatment, the better. You should be aware that scoliosis will remain with the child throughout his or her life. Take this opportunity to teach your child how to treat the body properly in terms of exercise, stretching, relaxation, and care in carrying (schoolbooks), posture, etc. The earlier a scoliosis patient is aware of how to best care for his or her body, the more benefit he or she will receive in later years. Scoliosis can present difficult psychological problems in a growing child. It is essential that the atmosphere be supportive and encouraging.

Young adults may also develop abnormal curves (at the end of their growth period) due to scoliosis that began in childhood and progressed. Older adults may develop osteoporosis and/or osteoarthritis. Possible consequences of this are changes in appearance (back looks crooked, hump may be visible), back pain, disabling lung disease, and increased stress on the heart.

To alleviate this, exercise gently and stretch as much as possible. Keep active and flexible to prevent stiffness and immobility.

INJURIES AND IRRITATIONS

Few active people, whether engaged in physical activity or under mental and emotional stress, get by without sustaining some form of injury or irritation. Some common injuries are

Strains. Injuries to tendons and muscles, occurring most frequently in the legs, strains are among the most common causes of back complaints. A strain can come from a muscle or tendon being too stretched, partially torn, or completely torn, usually requiring surgery.

Sprains are injuries to ligaments, which support joints. Again, they can result from muscles or tendons being stretched, partially torn, or completely torn. They are most common in ankles and knees.

Strains and sprains are best treated with RICE: rest, ice, compression, and elevation.

Stress injuries can result from overuse. Any activity, from jogging to playing a musical instrument, can cause a stress injury. There are two main types:

1. Stress fractures occur in the bones, most often below the knee and in the feet, but also in the vertebrae. Stress fractures usually heal by themselves, but activity must be limited as long as there is pain.
2. Tendonitis is an inflammation of the tendon, usually in the arms or legs. This is prevalent in musicians and athletes. Treatment involves limitation of activity, use of ice and heat, and anti-inflammatory drugs.

Bursitis. The bursa is a sac filled with fluid located between a tendon or muscle and a bone. It allows the tendon to glide smoothly. Bursitis, most common in the shoulders, elbows, hips, and knees, is an inflammation of the bursa. Like tendonitis, it is usually caused by overuse or disuse. Treatment is similar to tendonitis, except that the bursa may be injected with anti-inflammatory medication.

All of these injuries and irritations can be prevented by strengthening the muscles in the front of the body such as the abdominals and quadriceps and stretching the muscles of the back, back of thighs, etc. If you're engaged in a continuous activity, you should be aware of the responsibility to warm up, stretch, cool down, and generally start slowly and work up to maximum potential. Above all, don't work through pain; use it as a signal. Forget that old maxim, "No pain, no gain." In the long run, paying attention to pain will help avoid injuries.

ARTHRITIS

This is such a vast subject that volumes of books have been devoted to it. It is my intention here to give you a simple explanation of the causes and treatment of arthritis.

The word *arthritis* literally means "inflammation of a joint." However, the term is used to cover more than one hundred rheumatic diseases, some of which show no inflammation of joints. Sooner or later, everyone manifests some form of arthritis. It seems almost impossible to avoid, given the wear and tear of daily life. Although it is called America's number one crippler, it is not disabling (to the point of needing a wheelchair) to most people who have it. There is no cure, but there is relief. Because it affects everyone differently, it is essential that you learn as much as possible about your type to treat it in the most effective way.

Osteoarthritis (also called degenerative joint disease or osteoarthrosis) is the oldest known and most common disease in man, and every older adult has some form of it. It appears to be caused by overuse or misuse of joints, age, heredity, or obesity. It affects joint surfaces, cartilage, tendons, and joint capsules, and there is usually no inflammation. Although osteoarthritis can occur in any joint, some are more vulnerable than others—hips, knees, and cervical and lumbar spine. In the hands, it usually affects the last joints of the fingers (called Heberden's nodes, the bumps appear most frequently in women).

In the spine, osteoarthritis may also cause spinal stenosis, which is a narrowing of the openings in the vertebra usually caused by degenerative arthritis (also, occasionally, by injury, congenital defects, or spondylolisthesis—see page 184). Spinal stenosis may cause numbness or tingling in the arms, or sciatic-like pain in the legs when the nerve is pinched or stretched. Exercises to strengthen the abdominals and loosen the hip flexors and back extensors may help relieve this condition.

Rheumatoid arthritis can begin at any age and is less common. The ratio of degenerative joint arthritis to rheumatoid is six to one.

Whereas osteoarthritis is primarily "wear and tear," rheumatoid arthritis is an illness that may be associated with the autoimmune defense mechanisms. The cause is unknown, although there is a hereditary tendency and it may well be a virus. The membrane lining of the joint becomes swollen and visibly inflamed. Muscle stiffness occurs most frequently in the morning or after periods of inactivity, and seems to be aggravated by emotional stress. The pain and stiffness may last weeks, months, or years. In the worst cases, joints can become deformed and sufferers can become permanently crippled.

Ankylosing spondylitis (spinal arthritis) is even rarer, an inflammatory disease of the spine that causes fusion of the bones of the spine, hips, and shoulders. People who are completely bent over are probably suffering from this type. It occurs most frequently in men between the ages of sixteen and thirty-five and seems to be systemic in origin (which means it can be accompanied by fever, loss of appetite, and fatigue).

Fibrositis is characterized by pain in ligaments, tendons, and muscles. Chronic and usually intermittent but not deforming, it occurs most frequently in women between the ages of thirty-five and sixty. Stress, anxiety, and fatigue aggravate this condition; in fact, it may be related to a sleeping disorder. Sufferers of fibrositis develop sore spots, known as trigger points, most frequently along the upper back and neck.

Diagnosis for arthritis should be made by a doctor. Treatment varies greatly; it can range from aspirin, steroids, and anti-inflammatory drugs, to heat and cold, to gold salts, to corrective adjustments, manipulation, and surgery such as joint replacement. Rest and exercise are both important, and you must strike the right balance between the two. You must keep moving to keep the joints well oiled and to hydrate tissues. Knowledge of joint protection includes learning to use joints less stressfully and employ aids when necessary.

OVERWEIGHT

Overweight presents major problems for the back. Because of the strong connection between the abdominal and back muscles, extra weight in the abdominal area results in the body being pulled forward, forcing the back muscles to work harder. Even a few extra pounds in front can make the back have to counterbalance by exerting a strong force. This increases the curve of the lower back. In addition, excess weight puts tremendous pressure on joints—particularly knees, hips, and ankles. Also, if you're overweight, it's more difficult, physically and sometimes emotionally, to exercise, and exercise is essential to back health.

Even if you're heavy, you should still participate in an exercise program. There are really very few legitimate reasons for not losing weight, although one always can find several. Put away all your emotional considerations, such as how you look in a leotard or other exercise outfit. Just get in there and work. The results of proper exercise will put you in the right state to handle your weight problem, if you really want to.

Many overweight people are worried about drooping skin after weight loss. Certain exercises will help you lose weight but will not do much to get the body tighter or smaller. I had a student who lost thirty-nine pounds. The people in her office bet money on the number of pounds she had lost. All of them wrote down between eighty and eighty-five! They may have all lost, but she was the big winner.

When you do Callanetics, if you lose five pounds, you will look like you have lost ten to twenty; if you lose twenty, it will look like fifty.

We are all slaves to the scale. Again, numbers lie. As a nation, we have become totally obsessed with those tiny little numbers. We watch their daily journey up and down as though they had a life all their own. When you start to tighten up your body, you develop more muscle, and the muscle actually weighs more than fat. So we may become much smaller and tighter and yet not necessarily weigh less. If you want to watch numbers drop, watch the ones that say "size" on your clothes instead.

You cannot expect exercise alone to do the entire job. It's true that it can help to decrease your appetite. But you can't eat all kinds of fattening foods and then expect it to get you slim. You need a combination of sensible eating and a good exercise program.

CONSTIPATION

Constipation can aggravate or cause back pain. It should be corrected (with natural means, if possible) and avoided by the back patient. Also, in a chicken-and-egg situation, inactivity can bring on constipation, which in turn can aggravate back pain. You can avoid constipation by drinking lots of water and increasing the fiber in your diet; add raw bran to your food, if necessary.

Exercise plays a key role in preventing constipation. When I first started to teach, I would explain to students that they would experience more elimination each day as a result of doing Callanetics. This became a major topic of classroom conversation. When they discovered for themselves—no matter what their age—that what I said was true, they acted as though they just climbed Mt. Everest without ropes. Their excitement at the thought of never having to take another laxative was almost as much motivation for them to continue exercising as their new beautiful bodies!

OTHER CONDITIONS AND CIRCUMSTANCES

Spondylolisthesis is a slipped vertebra, usually caused by a break or separation of the back part of the vertebra. It may be due to some hereditary weakness, combined with long-term stress to the back such as extreme hyperextension of the lower back, as seen in teenage girls who are "powerhouse" gymnasts or ballet dancers. Most often, it affects the fifth lumbar vertebra and may cause pain when arching the back. You can do exercise to counteract the hyperextension (arching) such as the pelvic wave. Try to keep the lower back straight.

Recuperation from surgery. Nowhere are the advantages of exercise more pronounced than in the case of people who must undergo surgery and the resultant inactivity. It is well accepted that the more fit one is prior to a hospital stay or surgery, the quicker and more effective will be the recuperation. This fitness involves attitude, diet, and exercise, for the health of your musculature as well as your heart and lungs. Even in your hospital bed, you can do certain muscle-clenching and releasing exercises, then graduate, when you can move around, to more complex ones. Be sure to keep hands, feet, neck, and lower back as mobile as possible. Get moving as soon as your doctor allows you to. It has been said that you can lose as much as one fifth of your maximum muscle strength for every three days of being inactive. I agree totally. Start a gentle exercise program as quickly as you can after surgery—even if it means just walking up and down the hospital corridor.

Circulation; temperature changes. Blood circulation affects all parts of the body. And many factors affect circulation. For instance, such a simple procedure as a hot shower can change the way muscles feel. Cold can have varying effects as well. Sometimes people in pain feel particularly susceptible to cold. Or, if you're in a draft, you may end up with a stiff neck. On the other hand, ice is an effective treatment for soft-tissue injuries. Conditions such as arteriosclerosis and phlebitis affect blood flow, which in turn may create pain in your limbs.

If you chill easily or are one of those people who always needs to wear a sweater, you're probably suffering from poor circulation or low thyroid. Exercising is essential for poor circulation. A good indication of your need for this is the cramping of toes, which is common when you first begin an exercise program. As you progress, you'll notice that your circulation in general improves and the cramping ceases.

Sneezing and coughing. As much as possible, anticipate sneezing and coughing because the sudden, violent jar to the back may result in possible serious effects. Stop whatever you're doing, sit or stand straight, try to bend your knees, curl up your pelvis and tighten your buttocks (pelvic wave); support your abdomen with your hands.

14.

Other Ways and Means to Relieve Back Symptoms

While I was working on this book, my studio floor became one bumpy carpet of gadgets, pillows, backrests, massagers, etc. The majority of them were wonderful, except for most of the electric massagers—which were pathetic.

A few years ago, it was a rarity to see an ad for back helpers in magazines, catalogs, or on television. Now it seems that everywhere you look there's something new designed to help a bad back. In this chapter you'll find a Resources section that lists companies from which you can obtain catalogs that offer back "helpers." They are all companies I have tried and recommend.

What follows is a brief discussion of some other kinds of helpers.

BEDS/MATTRESSES

Considering how much time you spend sleeping or just lying down, the choice of a bed is a major one. A comfortable bed is one of the most important pieces of furniture you purchase in your lifetime. Just as no two bodies are alike, there can be no rules about which is the best bed. Some people prefer the hardest of surfaces (even sleeping on the floor), whereas others must have something soft beneath them.

A girlfriend of mine had a special mattress made exclusively for her back. She paid two thousand dollars for it. She despised it. I, on the other hand, had one with bumps, lumps, and probably broken springs. We decided to switch. She loves that embarrassing mattress, and I'm thrilled with hers—particularly after I covered it with my new feather mattress.

Naturally, lumpy, sagging mattresses are not the ideal choice, but aside from that, you have free reign. *Comfort* is the key word. Some of the broad categories of beds and helpers are:

Adjustable beds. Both the head and foot on some models can be raised and lowered to several positions (similar to hospital beds); controls are independent to enable one person to adjust his or her side without disturbing the other.

"Orthopedic" mattresses. Depending on the brand, these will have different names. This is really confusing. How is one supposed to choose a mattress—lie on it for twenty seconds in the store, feeling really stupid? Who knows the difference between a "Kealy pealy," "Ostomedic," "Bedic," and "Electricmedic"? What they have in common is a design that is supposedly good for the back; they come in a variety of firmnesses (which, of course, is also confusing, as some say soft is best, others hard.)

Waterbeds. Some people with lower back problems swear by these. Some can also be heated for additional comfort.

Boards. These are placed under the mattress and over the springs to make the surface firmer. (Sometimes placing the mattress on the floor will accomplish the same purpose, but then what do you do with your bed?) They can be purchased or made to order; some even fold for greater portability.

Mattress pads. Where do you begin? Some say wool is the best material because it helps control body temperature, relieve points of pressure on the back, lessen tossing and turning, and is excellent for arthritis. Others say nothing compares to a thick, convoluted foam pad because moisture, heat, and friction are reduced. There are also electric heating mattress pads that you can adjust to any temperature. There's a contoured foam pad that actually massages you as you sleep. And then there's down, which is what's in my feather mattress. I place it on top of the mattress and it feels absolutely luxurious. Somehow, I don't wake up with as many kinks as before.

Futons (cotton mattresses). These have been borrowed from the Orient and have become very popular. They come in a selection of thicknesses, and can be rolled up during the day and placed directly on the floor or on a frame for sleeping; they convert from a couch to a bed with the slightest effort.

PILLOWS/NECK RESTS

There is a wide variety of pillows for supporting the neck, shoulders, and back. Here are some broad classifications:

Wedge (triangular) shaped pillows eliminate the need for multiple pillows, are excellent for exercising (see Three Stages, page 113), serve as back rests, and can also be used to elevate knees.

Cervical (neck) rolls can be used to support and maintain neck curve instead of, or with, a pillow. Some pillows are available with neck rolls sewn in; there's even a pillowcase for your favorite pillow with a removable neck roll.

Inflatable pillows for traveling fold into pocket-size.

Crescent or U-shaped pillows for traveling or sitting snap around neck and help eliminate kinks in neck while sleeping in cars, etc.

Convoluted thick foam pillows come with or without depressions for head.

Orthopedic pillows have combination firm and soft sides.

Massage pillows vibrate, are shockproof, and some are even waterproof for use in the bath.

To obtain catalogues, see Resources, page 190.

GRAVITY INVERSION EQUIPMENT

This is a fancy name for any equipment that has you hanging upside down or tilted at an angle. The reasoning behind gravity inversion is that because it takes weight off the legs, it decompresses the spine and stretches the lower back. Some people swear that defying gravity may be one way to delay aging. The mildest version of this is a slant board, where the feet are up and the head down at whatever angle you choose. Supposedly, a slant board straightens the spine and, because the blood flows from the feet toward the head, reduces swelling in the legs. There are exercise programs that employ a slant board (I am absolutely opposed to doing abdominal exercises on one), but in most cases it's used for relaxation.

More complex equipment has people hanging upside down from specially fastened boots or controlling the angle at which they hang. There are several variations on that theme, and I'm not thrilled with any of them.

Not everyone is a candidate for gravity inversion—even for slant boards. If you have hypertension or any other condition that might be aggravated by blood rushing to your head, don't do it. Even if you're healthy, be careful getting off a slant board. If you do it abruptly, you're likely to become dizzy.

HOME EXERCISE EQUIPMENT

There is an enormous selection of machines you can buy to exercise in the comfort of your home. Most of it is elaborate and expensive, such as equipment that simulates an entire gym. Advantages to exercise machines at home are convenience in terms of time, weather, and privacy. It seems to me that a person must be rather well-motivated to use them on a regular basis.

Some home exercisers worth noting include a cushioned mini-trampoline on which to jog that reduces the impact on knees and back; a folding treadmill; a machine that simulates cross-country skiing; and—my absolute favorite—an exercise bicycle weighing a mere 7½ pounds and small enough to tuck anywhere because it consists only of foot pedals. As a seat you use your own chair! You can watch television and get a workout at the same time. Isn't that ingenious?

HOT/COLD

Nothing seems to cause more emotional opinions about what's better for back discomfort: heat or cold. This even includes doctors and other specialists. I myself love heat, and the thought of ice on my lower back makes me turn blue and feel like tensing.

Heat. At the first sign of back pain, people usually think "heat" and run for the heating pad. Alternatives include hot water bottles, hot moist towels, and hot baths. Some people even install saunas or whirlpools to help their back, as well as for general relaxation. Whichever method you choose, it's important to keep these points in mind:

- Heat does relieve discomfort and is certainly relaxing. But because it brings blood to the area, it may be prohibited in some cases where inflamed muscles are already congested, or where there is pain in the nerve. For instance, heat may make sciatica worse.
- Don't overdo it, either in length of time or degree of temperature. Never use heat more than ten or fifteen minutes without taking a rest. Regarding temperature, a bath, hot towel, or hot water bottle are probably preferable to a heating pad because the latter can become too hot. Always wrap a hot water bottle or heating pad in a towel. A half-filled hot water bottle placed between the shoulder blades or on your lower back feels wonderful.
- I prefer moist heat because it penetrates better and doesn't dehydrate the muscles. If you use a heating pad, place a moist washcloth or towel over your skin and then place the pad on top (be sure that it is insulated properly; don't risk any electrical shocks on top of your spasms—it will feel as if your heart is jumping out of your body!)

The following are some unique helpers using heat:

Pads for neck, spine, knee, shoulders, and even sinuses that electrically produce their own moisture from the air.

An electrical heating cover that fits over a chair back and seat.

Infrared heat devices that can be used at home. These devices are held in the hand and applied to the neck, back, knees, etc.

Heat massagers that combine vibrators with electrically controlled heat.

Hydrocolators, canvas pads filled with a substance that retains heat when warmed by boiling in water, can be used on the back and neck; portable moist heat packs are reusable and will heat by simply pushing a "button" inside the pack.

Ice. This method has always been prescribed immediately after an injury such as a sprain to reduce the swelling. The American College of Sports Medicine recommends RICE—rest, ice, compression, elevation. Now there seems to be further interest in ice for relieving spasms, as well as to keep blood away from the area, thereby reducing inflammation. You can use something as simple as ice cubes in a sealproof plastic bag, or an ice pack (kept in the freezer for emergencies); or try some of the more sophisticated items listed below. As with heat, always cover ice with a towel before applying it to the skin. You could actually get frostbite if you don't! Ice should be applied ten minutes on, ten minutes off for as long as two hours for an acute injury, or two or three times a day for chronic pain.

Some other helpers for cold treatments are:
Mineral ice or some other form of gel that is rubbed into skin and feels cold as it penetrates deep into muscles.

Wraps that can be placed on areas such as neck and knees. They contain a gel that can be made cold (or heated). You can wear these wraps and still move around freely.

Combination of hot and cold. This is considered by some to be far more effective than either hot or cold alone. The most commonly used method is alternating heat with cold, ten minutes of each with ten minutes rest in between. If you have a condition such as tendonitis and you continue doing an activity (playing a musical instrument, for example), the accepted treatment is heat before the activity (to warm up) and ice afterward.

It's a good idea to ask a specialist for an opinion before using either heat or ice or the combination.

See page 190 for information on ordering catalogs featuring these items.

PAINKILLERS

It may be as surprising to you as it was to me to find out that drugs are the most often used treatment for back pain. These can take many forms, from over-the-counter aspirin (hardly as harmless as we used to think) to muscle relaxants, antiinflammatory drugs, and tranquilizers (the most widely used painkiller is also a popular tranquilizer). You can swallow pills or be injected either directly into a muscle or at a trigger point.

There is no question that the pain of an acute spasm can be

excruciating and that it is perfectly normal for someone to reach for the quickest relief possible. The problem with most painkillers is that they do just that—and little else. They are temporary and do not act on the cause or provide long-term relief of the problem. Many of them act as nerve blocks (the same principle as dental anesthetic), interrupting the signal being sent from the painful area to the brain. (Since you don't feel pain until the signal reaches the brain, these blocks can work. So does acupuncture, which works on the same principle; see pages 152–153.)

In addition to drugs being only temporary, there are other difficulties. First is the obvious question of side effects and possible addiction, which is common with many drugs prescribed for physical conditions. But, more specific to the back is the issue of the effect of masking pain. If you're in pain, the amount of activity you can do is usually severely limited. And this may be just what may be required. But if the pain is blocked, you run the risk of doing further injury to yourself because you don't "feel" enough. Also, drugs can sometimes mask serious injuries.

Here's something I find quite startling. The results of a popular survey done among back sufferers indicated only about 30 percent received even temporary relief from drugs (no drug proved effective in the long term).

The option to take some sort of painkiller is a strictly personal matter. However, it's wise to weigh all the considerations before making that choice, and, naturally, to consult with your practitioner.

RESOURCES

The following is a list of companies that distribute aids for the back, some of which I have tried and would recommend. They will send catalogs and other information on request.

Comfortably Yours
61 W. Hunter Avenue
Maywood, NJ 07607
(201) 368-0400

The Sharper Image
650 Davis Street
San Francisco, CA 94111
1-800-344-4444

Hammacher Schlemmer
147 E. 57th Street
New York, NY 10022
(212) 421-9000

Vermont Country Store
P.O. Box 3000
Manchester Center, VT 05255-3000
(802) 362-4667

Markline
14 Jewel Drive
Wilmington, MA 01887-9988
(617) 658-0760

Wahl Clipper Corp.
2900 N. Locust Street
P.O. Box 578
Sterling, IL 61081-0578
(815) 625-6525

Index

abdominal exercises, 57, 109–122
  dangerous, 146–147
Achilles tendon, 38, 39
acupuncturists, 152–153
aerobic dancing, 150–151
aging, 166–168, 173
airplane travel, 70–71, 74–82
Alexander technique, 156
anatomy, 169–174
arm exercises, 31, 46, 76
  underarm, 28, 98–99, 100–103
  upper arm, 26, 27
arthritis, 181–182

back, 169–174
  exercises for, 51–58, 77, 78, 79–81, 131
  pain, 175–184
back schools, 158
beds, 64, 185–186
bending, 69, 176
bones, 169–171
breathing, 25, 86, 98, 99
bursitis, 155, 180–181
buttocks, exercises for, 29, 44, 57, 121–125, 131
  dangerous, 147–148

Callanetics, three stages of, 83–137
calves, exercises for, 38, 39, 128
carrying, 66, 67–69, 70–71
cars, 71, 74–82
cartilage, 172
chest, exercises for, 26, 27, 29–30, 57
children, 164–166
chiropractors, 153–154, 156
circulation, 184
close quarters, exercises for, 74–82
constipation, 183

dangerous exercises, 139–148
doctors, 149, 151–152

everyday activities, 59–71
everyday exercises, 73–82
exercise machines, 187, 188
exercise programs, 150–151, 156

family practitioners, 152
feet, 47–50, 59, 155
Feldenkrais, 156
fibrositis, 182
fractures, 180

gravity inversion equipment, 187

hamstrings, exercises for, 39, 40–42, 127–128, 141–142
  dangerous, 141–142
hanging exercises, 45, 178
hip exercises, 29, 33, 57, 121–125, 131, 177

injuries, 180–181, 189
  preventing, 18, 23, 24, 86, 126, 140, 151, 181

Jin Shin Jyutsu, 155–156
joints, 172, 173

kinesiology, 156
knees, dangerous exercises and, 141, 143

leg exercises, 77
  dangerous, 146–148
lifting, 66–67, 71, 176
ligaments, 173, 180
lordosis (swayback), 121, 155, 179

massage, 154–155, 164–165
mattresses, 64, 185–186
movement therapists, 156
muscles, 174, 180

neck exercises, 29–30, 31, 38, 39, 43–44, 46, 75, 94–98
  dangerous, 144–145
nerves, 173, 174

occupational therapists, 154
orthopedists, 151–152
orthotics, 50
osteopaths, 152
overweight, 166, 182–183

pain, 17, 85, 140, 160, 175–184
  relief from, 83, 84, 189–190
pain clinics, 158
pelvic rotations, 50, 132–135
pelvic wave, 19, 50, 88–93, 178, 184
physiatrists, 152
physical education, 165–166
physical therapists, 154
positive thinking, 18, 25, 85, 86, 159–163, 167
posture, 47, 59, 94, 98–99, 161, 165, 174
psoas, 32–33, 128, 179
pulling and pushing, 69–70, 71

Reiki, 155–156
relaxing, 58, 86, 110

resistance equipment, 148
resources, 190

sciatica, 155, 175–176
sciatic nerve, 173
scoliosis, 155, 177–180
shiatsu, 155
shoes, 48–49, 59, 164
shoulder blades, stretches for between, 30, 31, 38, 118
shoulder exercises, 26, 27, 29–30, 46, 76, 78, 81–82
  dangerous, 144–145
sitting, 59, 61–63, 71
slant boards, 187
sleeping, 63–64, 90, 185
spasm, 86, 161–162, 189–190
  exercises for, 19–21, 57
spinal stenosis, 181
spine, 47–48, 167, 169–174, 177–180
  dangerous exercises and, 143–144
  exercises for, 29–30, 31, 38, 39, 44, 46, 57
spondylolisthesis, 181, 184
sports medicine doctors, 152
standing, 59–60
strains and sprains, 180
stress, 162–163
stretching, 23–46, 126
surgery, 179, 184
swayback (lordosis), 63, 89, 95, 121, 140, 155, 179

t'ai chi chuan, 156–157
tendons, 173, 180
thighs, front, exercises for, 32, 128, 129–130
  dangerous, 142–143
thighs, inner, exercises for, 34–37, 39, 111, 136–137
thighs, outer, exercises for, 29, 44, 57, 121–125
Touch for Health, 155

vertebrae, 169, 170–171, 176, 184

waist exercises, 31, 104–108
  dangerous, 145–146
walking, 59, 60–61
warming up, 25, 87, 90
weight lifting, 148, 172

YMCA-YWCA, 156
yoga, 144, 157

12 MONTHS ON
THE NEW YORK TIMES
BESTSELLER LIST!

AS FEATURED ON
NATIONAL TELEVISION AND ON
THE BEST-SELLING VIDEO!

THE ASTONISHING DEEP-MUSCLE
EXERCISE THAT CAN GIVE YOU
A PERFECT FIGURE

10 YEARS YOUNGER
IN 10 HOURS

Callanetics

by CALLAN PINCKNEY

70261-4/$12.50 U.S./$15.00 Can